DEJA REVIEW™

Pharmacology

NOTICE

Medicine is an ever-changing science. As new research and clinical experience broaden our knowledge, changes in treatment and drug therapy are required. The authors and the publisher of this work have checked with sources believed to be reliable in their efforts to provide information that is complete and generally in accord with the standards accepted at the time of publication. However, in view of the possibility of human error or changes in medical sciences, neither the authors nor the publisher nor any other party who has been involved in the preparation or publication of this work warrants that the information contained herein is in every respect accurate or complete, and they disclaim all responsibility for any errors or omissions or for the results obtained from use of the information contained in this work. Readers are encouraged to confirm the information contained herein with other sources. For example and in particular, readers are advised to check the product information sheet included in the package of each drug they plan to administer to be certain that the information contained in this work is accurate and that changes have not been made in the recommended dose or in the contraindications for administration. This recommendation is of particular importance in connection with new or infrequently used drugs.

DEJA REVIEW™

Pharmacology

Second Edition

Jessica A. Gleason, M.D.

Stony Brook University
B.S. Pharmacology with Departmental Honors
Stony Brook, New York

School of Medicine
Stony Brook University Medical Center
Doctor of Medicine
Stony Brook, New York Class of 2010

Beth Israel Deaconess Medical Center
Department of Anesthesiology
Harvard Medical School
Boston, MA

St. Vincent Hospital
Department of Medicine
Worcester, MA

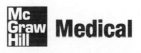

New York   Chicago   San Francisco   Lisbon   London   Madrid   Mexico City
Milan   New Delhi   San Juan   Seoul   Singapore   Sydney   Toronto

Déjà Review™: Pharmacology, Second Edition

6 7 8 9 0   DOC/DOC   14 13

ISBN 978-0-07-162729-0
MHID 0-07-162729-4

This book was set in Palatino by Glyph International.

The editors were Kirsten Funk and Karen G. Edmonson.

The production supervisor was Catherine H. Saggese.

Project management was provided by Somya Rustagi, Glyph International.

RR Donnelley was printer and binder.

This book is printed on acid-free paper.

Library of Congress Cataloging-in-Publication Data

Gleason, Jessica A.
    Deja review. Pharmacology / Jessica A. Gleason.—2nd ed.
        p. ; cm.—(Deja review)
    Other title: Pharmacology
    Includes bibliographical references and index.
    ISBN-13: 978-0-07-162729-0 (pbk. : alk. paper)
    ISBN-10: 0-07-162729-4 (pbk. : alk. paper)   1. Pharmacology—Examinations, questions, etc.   I. Title. II. Title: Pharmacology.   III. Series: Deja review.
    [DNLM: 1. Pharmacological Phenomena—Examination Questions.   2. Drug Therapy—Examination Questions.   3. Pharmaceutical Preparations—Examination Questions.   QV 18.2 G554d   2010]
    RM301.13.Y68   2010
    615'.1076—dc22
                                                                    2010018582

This book is dedicated to Adam. Your confidence in me has enriched my career, and your love for me has enriched my life.
—Jessica A. Gleason

Contents

Faculty Reviewer

Miguel Berrios, Ph.D.
Department of Pharmacology
School of Medicine
State University of New York
Stony Brook, New York

Student Reviewers

Joe Bart
Lake Erie College of Osteopathic Medicine
Bradenton Division
Class of 2008

Rosalyn Pham
University of Washington
School of Medicine
Class of 2008

Alexis M. Dallara
SUNY Downstate
College of Medicine
Class of 2009

Preface

The *Deja Review* series is a unique resource that has been designed to allow you to review the essential facts and determine your level of knowledge on the subjects tested on Step 1 of the United States Medical Licensing Examination (USMLE). The format of this book is highly beneficial to aid one's understanding of the subject of pharmacology for several reasons. The breadth of the subject material could quickly become over-whelming without some sort of organizational framework, provided concisely and coherently in this book. The question/answer format allows for quick reviews of famil-iar concepts, and moreover is conducive to repetition, which, above all else, will be nec-essary to master this subject. The new, expanded clinical vignettes section now follow each chapter in this edition to allow you to test that you are able to integrate the knowl-edge you have obtained and ensure your grasp on the material extends beyond rote memorization. A great effort has been made in this edition to expand emphasis on clin-ical application and to make necessary updates to this ever evolving realm of medicine.

ORGANIZATION

All concepts are presented in a question and answer format that covers key facts on commonly tested topics in medical pharmacology. The first chapter introduces the basic principles of the subject. Then the chapters move through defined subtopics within pharmacology. A series of vignettes follows most chapters. These vignettes are meant to be representative of the types of questions tested on national licensing exams to help you further evaluate your understanding of the material presented in the chapter. The compact, condensed design of the book is conducive to studying on the go, especially during any downtime throughout your day.

This question and answer format has several important advantages:

- It provides a rapid, straightforward way for you to assess your strengths and weaknesses.
- It allows you to efficiently review and commit to memory a large body of information.
- It serves as a quick, last-minute review of high-yield facts.

At the end of each chapter, you will find clinical vignettes that expose you to the pro-totypic presentation of diseases classically tested on the USMLE Step 1. These board-style questions put the basic science into a clinical context, allowing you apply the facts you have just reviewed in a clinical scenario.

HOW TO USE THIS BOOK

Remember, this text is not intended to replace comprehensive textbooks, course packs, or lectures. It is simply intended to serve as a supplement to your studies during your medical pharmacology course and Step 1 preparation. This text was contributed to by a number of medical students to represent the core topics tested on course examinations and Step 1. You may use the book to quiz yourself or classmates on topics covered in recent lectures and clinical case discussions. A bookmark is included so that you can easily cover up the answers as you work through each chapter.

However you choose to study, I hope you find this resource helpful throughout your preparation for course examinations, the USMLE Step 1, and other national licensing exams.

Jessica Gleason

Acknowledgments

The author would like to thank Miguel Berrios, Ph.D., Kirsten Funk, Editor, and Somya Rustagi, Project Manager for their invaluable contributions to this text and their efforts in making this a useful resource for students.

CHAPTER 1

Basic Principles

Basic principles are often perceived as the most challenging aspect of learning pharmacology. While possibly conceptually difficult, this subject is absolutely key to gain understanding how medications exert their effects and side effects. While licensing exams may not stress basic principles in their pure form, this topic is at the core of many pharmacology questions that may appear in these examinations. Therefore, a strong knowledge of basic principles will help you with your study of pharmacology, and throughout your medical career.

PHARMACOKINETICS

Define the following terms:

Pharmacokinetics

Field of study that deals with time required for drug absorption, distribution in the body, metabolism, and method of excretion. In short, it is the body's effect on the drug.

Volume of distribution (V_d)

The apparent volume in the body available to contain the drug. Formula: $V_d = \text{Dose/Plasma Drug Concentration}$

Is V_d a physiologic value?

No

$V_d = dose / [plasma drug]$

$$\dfrac{dose}{[plasma]\ of\ drug}$$

1

Is V_d an absolute value for any given drug?

No

Clearance (Cl)

Volume of blood cleared of the drug per unit time; Cl = Rate of elimination of drug/plasma drug concentration; Total Body Cl = $Cl_{hepatic}$ + Cl_{renal} + $Cl_{pulmonary}$ + Cl_{other}

Half-life ($t_{1/2}$)

$$\frac{.693 \cdot V_d}{Cl}$$

Time required for plasma concentration of drug to decrease by one-half after absorption and distribution are complete; $t_{1/2} = (0.693 \times V_d)/(Cl)$

Bioavailability (F)

The fraction of (active) drug that reaches the systemic circulation/site of action after administration by any route; F = $(AUC_{po})/(AUC_{iv})$, where AUC_{po} and AUC_{iv} are the extravascular and intravenous areas under the plasma concentration versus time curves, respectively

Steady state (C_{ss})

Steady state is reached when the rate of drug influx into the body = the rate of drug elimination out of the body; C_{ss} = plasma concentration of drug at steady state

How much drug is left after two half-lives?

25%

How much drug is left after three half-lives?

12.5%

During constant infusion, what percent of steady state is reached after one half-life?

50%

During constant infusion, what percent of steady state is reached after two half-lives?

75%

During constant infusion, what percent of steady state is reached after three half-lives?

87.5%

During constant infusion, what percent of steady state is reached after four half-lives?

94%

Give the equation for the following terms:

[Plasm] of drug @ stany svc

Infusion rate (k_0)

$k_0 = Cl \times C_{ss}$

Loading dose (LD)

$LD = (V_d \times C_{ss})/(F)$; for examination purposes, F is usually 1

Maintenance dose (MD)

$(Cl \times C_{ss} \times \tau)/(F)$, where τ (tao) is the dosing interval

Clearance (Cl)

$Cl = K \times V_d$, where K is the elimination constant

Volume of distribution (V_d)

$V_d = (LD)/(C_{ss})$

Half-life ($t_{1/2}$)

$t_{1/2} = (0.693)/(K)$ or $(0.693 \times V_d)/(Cl)$

What happens to the steady state concentration of a drug if the infusion rate is doubled?

Steady state concentration is also doubled; remember that dose and concentration are directly proportional (linear kinetics); $C_{ss} \times k_0/Cl$

If there is no active secretion or reabsorption, then renal clearance (Cl_{renal}) is equal to what?

Glomerular filtration rate (GFR)

If a drug is protein bound, then Cl_{renal} is equal to what?

GFR × free fraction (of drug)

What happens to the LD in patients with impaired renal or hepatic function?   *K- maithe dage.*

Stays the same

What happens to the MD in patients with impaired renal or hepatic function?

Decreases

For each of the following statements, state whether it refers to zero-order elimination or first-order elimination?

Rate of elimination is constant, regardless of concentration

Zero-order elimination

Plasma concentration decreases exponentially with time

First-order elimination

Rate of elimination is proportional to the drug concentration

First-order elimination

Plasma concentration decreases linearly with time

Zero-order elimination

Rate of elimination is independent of concentration

Zero-order elimination

Rate of elimination is dependent on concentration

First-order elimination *(biphsc)*

What are some examples of drugs/ substances that undergo zero-order elimination?

Acetylsalicylic acid (Aspirin, ASA) at high/toxic concentrations; phenytoin; ethanol

Describe the following types of metabolism:

Phase I metabolism

Metabolism that generally yields more polar, water-soluble metabolites (may still be active); enzyme activity decreases with patient's age

Phase II metabolism

Metabolism that generally yields very polar, inactive metabolites (renally excreted); enzyme activity does not decrease with patient's age

Phase I (microsomal) metabolism involves what types of reactions?

Oxidation; reduction; hydrolysis (carried out by cytochrome P-450 enzymes)

Phase II (nonmicrosomal) metabolism involves what types of reactions?

Glucuronidation; acetylation; sulfation; amidation; glutathione conjugation

Give examples of drugs that undergo phase II metabolism:

Isoniazid (INH), morphine, 6-mercaptopurine, acetaminophen

What are the potential consequences of phase I oxidation reactions with regard to drug activity and elimination?

Drug activity may or may not change (no rule, ie, potentially dangerous outcome). Drug elimination is usually increased due to greater water solubility.

What are the potential consequences of phase II reactions with regard to drug activity and elimination?

Drug products of phase II reactions are usually inactive and their renal elimination is enhanced.

Where are cytochrome P-450 enzymes found?

Smooth endoplasmic reticulum of cells in mainly the liver, but also found in the gastrointestinal (GI) tract, kidney, and lungs

Explain what each type of the following clinical phases in drug development is trying to accomplish?

Phase I

Safety in healthy individuals; drug pharmacokinetics

Phase II

Efficacy in diseased individuals (small scale trials, single- or double-blind)

Phase III

Efficacy in diseased individuals (large scale trials, mainly double-blind)

Phase IV

Postmarketing surveillance (monitored release)

At what point during drug development is an investigational new drug (IND) application filed?

Before phase I

At what point during drug development is a new drug application (NDA) filed?

After phase III (and before phase IV)

What does the term bioequivalence mean?

When comparing two formulations of the same compound, they are said to be bioequivalent to each other if they have the same bioavailability and the same rate of absorption.

What is the first-pass effect?

After oral administration, many drugs are absorbed intact from the small intestine and transported first via the portal system to the liver, where they undergo extensive metabolism, therefore usually decreasing the bioavailability of certain oral medications.

How many liters are in each of the following compartments of an average adult human?

Blood

5 L

Plasma

3 L

Total body water (TBW)

42 L (avg. 70 kg man × 60%. For women 50% of mass [body weight] in kg is body water due to lower lean muscle mass and higher fat content [adipose tissue]).

What is the most common plasma protein that drugs bind to?

Albumin

Displacing a drug that is bound to plasma protein(s), for example, albumin, will increase its what?

Its free fraction (therefore may possibly increase the risk of toxicity because the plasma concentration of active drug has been increased, yet depending on the drug, an increase in free fraction may actually increase its metabolism because more drug is available to metabolizing enzymes)

For each of the following mechanisms of membrane transport, state if energy is required, if a carrier is required, and if the system is saturable?

Passive diffusion

No energy required; no carrier; not saturable (proportional to concentration gradient)

Facilitated diffusion

No energy required; carrier required; saturable

Active transport

Against concentration/electrical gradient, therefore energy required; carrier required; saturable

The permeation of drugs across cellular membranes is dependent on what drug properties and (local) circumstances?

Drug solubility; drug concentration gradient; drug ionization; surface area; vascularity

Acidification of urine will increase renal elimination of what types of drugs?

Weak bases (ionized form of drug, BH^+) will be trapped in the renal tubules and thus excreted in the urine.

Acidification of urine will decrease renal elimination of what types of drugs?

Weak acids (nonionized, HA, form of a drug) can cross membranes.

Alkalinization of urine will increase renal elimination of what types of drugs?

Weak acids (ionized, A^-, form of a drug) will be trapped in the renal tubules and thus excreted in the urine.

Alkalinization of urine will decrease renal elimination of what types of drugs?

Weak bases (nonionized, B, form of a drug) can cross membranes.

What agents are used to acidify urine?	NH_4Cl; high dose of vitamin C
What agents are used to alkalinize urine?	$NaHCO_3$; acetazolamide
Give an example of a weakly acidic drug:	Acetylsalicylic acid (ASA); barbiturates
Give an example of a weakly basic drug:	Amphetamines
Give examples of drugs metabolized by each of the following cytochrome P-450 enzymes metabolizes:	
CYP 1A2	Caffeine; ciprofloxacin; theophylline; R-warfarin
CYP 2C9	Ibuprofen; naproxen; phenytoin; S-warfarin
CYP 2C19	Diazepam; omeprazole
CYP 2D6	Codeine; dextromethorphan; fluoxetine; haloperidol; loratadine; metoprolol; paroxetine; risperidone; thioridazine; venlafaxine
CYP 2E1	Ethanol; INH; acetaminophen (at high doses)
CYP 3A4 (50%-60% of all therapeutically used drugs are metabolized via CYP 3A4)	Alprazolam; carbamazepine; cyclosporine; diltiazem; erythromycin; fluconazole; itraconazole; ketoconazole; lidocaine; lovastatin; midazolam; nifedipine; quinidine; simvastatin; tacrolimus; verapamil
Give examples of drugs and herbal extracts that generally induce cytochrome P-450 enzymes:	Phenobarbital; nicotine; rifampin; phenytoin; carbamazepine; St. John's wort; chronic ethanol consumption
Give examples of drugs and foods that generally inhibit cytochrome P-450 enzymes:	Erythromycin; ketoconazole; ciprofloxacin; quinidine; cimetidine; omeprazole; ritonavir; chloramphenicol; acute alcohol intoxication, grapefruit juice

The following graph depicts what type of elimination?

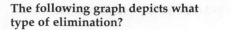
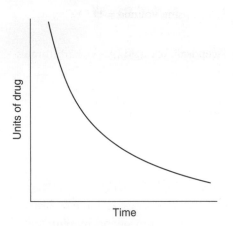
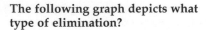

First-order elimination

The following graph depicts what type of elimination?

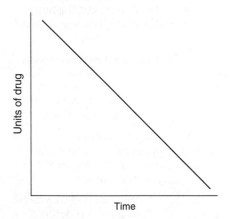

Zero-order elimination

Intracellular volume (ICV) makes up what fraction of TBW?	2/3 (ICV = 2/3 TBW)
Extracellular volume (ECV) makes up what fraction of TBW?	1/3 (ECV = 1/3 TBW)

Interstitial volume makes up what fraction of ECV?	2/3 (interstitial volume = 2/3 ECV)
Plasma volume makes up what fraction of ECV?	1/3 (plasma volume = 1/3 ECV)
What type of elimination involves a constant *fraction* of drug eliminated per unit time?	First-order elimination
What type of elimination involves a constant *amount* of drug eliminated per unit time?	Zero-order elimination

PHARMACODYNAMICS

Define the following terms:

Pharmacodynamics (PD)	Field of study that deals with the relationship between plasma concentration of a drug and the body response obtained to that drug; in short, the drug's effect on the body
Affinity	Ability of a drug to bind to a receptor; on a graded dose-response curve, the nearer the curve is to the y axis, the greater the affinity (affinity deals with drugs acting on the same receptor)
Efficacy	How well a drug produces a pharmacological response; on a graded dose-response curve, the height of the curve represents the efficacy
Potency	The amount of drug required to obtain a desired effect; on a graded dose-response curve, the nearer the curve is to the y axis, the greater the potency
Will the curves for two drugs acting on the same receptor be parallel or nonparallel to each other on a graded dose-response curve?	Parallel

Will the curves for two drugs acting on different receptors be parallel or nonparallel to each other on a graded dose-response curve?

Nonparallel

For the graph below, which drug has greater potency?

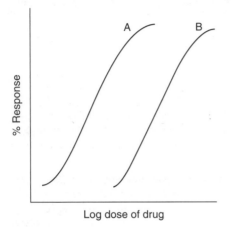

Drug A

For the graph below, which drug has greater efficacy?

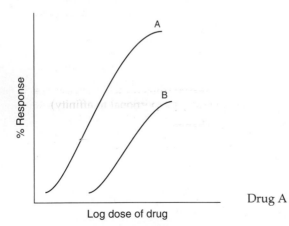

Drug A

Define the following terms:

Agonist	A drug that binds to a receptor, alters its conformation, and activates that receptor's function
Full agonist	An agonist capable of producing a maximal response
Partial agonist	An agonist incapable of producing a maximal response; less efficacious than a full agonist
Antagonist	A drug that binds to a receptor and prevents activation of a receptor
Competitive antagonist	An antagonist that competes with an agonist for the same receptor site; graded dose-response curve will be shifted to the right (parallel) thus decreasing the agonist's potency (and affinity); maximal response will not be affected

(no Δ max respse)
↓ ptncy (right shft

Noncompetitive antagonist	An antagonist that acts at a different site from the agonist, yet still prevents the agonist from activating its receptor; potency not affected; maximal response will be decreased; causes a nonparallel shift to the right on a graded dose-response curve

(↓ max respne
no Δ in ptncy)

What happens when a partial agonist is added in the presence of a full agonist?	The response of the full agonist is reduced; partial agonist is acting as an antagonist.

How does a competitive antagonist affect the following?

Affinity ($1/K_m$) of agonist	Decreased (thus K_m will increase as it is inversely proportional to affinity)
Maximal response (V_{max}) of agonist	No change

How does a noncompetitive antagonist affect the following?

Affinity ($1/K_m$) of agonist	No change
Maximal response (V_{max}) of agonist	Decreased

What type of antagonism does the following graph represent?

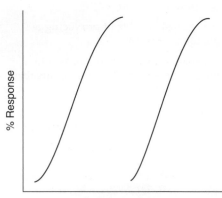

Competitive antagonism

What type of antagonism does the following graph represent?

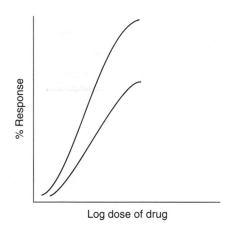

Noncompetitive antagonism

What type of antagonism does the following graph represent?

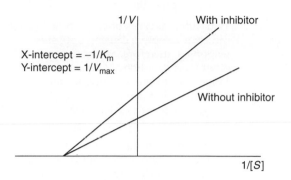

X-intercept = $-1/K_m$
Y-intercept = $1/V_{max}$

1/V|

With inhibitor

Without inhibitor

1/[S]

Noncompetitive antagonism

What type of antagonism does the following graph represent?

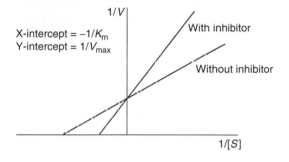

1/V|

X-intercept = $-1/K_m$
Y-intercept = $1/V_{max}$

With inhibitor

Without inhibitor

1/[S]

Competitive antagonism

Will increasing the dose of an agonist completely reverse the effect of a competitive antagonist?   Yes

Will increasing the dose of an agonist completely reverse the effect of a noncompetitive antagonist?   No

Define the following terms:

Pharmacologic antagonism	Antagonist and agonist compete for the same receptor site.
Physiologic antagonism	Two different types of agonists acting at different receptors causing opposite responses, therefore, antagonizing each other (acetylcholine [ACh] activating an M receptor to cause bradycardia is antagonized by norepinephrine [NE] acting at a β-receptor to cause tachycardia)
Chemical antagonism	Response to a drug is antagonized by another compound that binds directly to the effector drug (digoxin is antagonized by digoxin immune F_{ab} [Digibind] which binds directly to digoxin and not its receptor)
Potentiation	When one agonist enhances the action of another compound (benzodiazepines and barbiturates potentiate the effect of gamma-aminobutyric acid (GABA) on its receptor); graded dose-response curve is shifted to the left
What is a quantal (cumulative) dose-response curve?	Curve showing the percentage of a population responding to a given drug effect versus dose of drug given (or log of dose); allows you to visualize intersubject variability regarding drug response in graph form
What is ED_{50}?	Estimation of the effective dose in 50% of a population; the dose at which 50% of the population will respond to the drug
Can you obtain the ED_{50} from a graded (quantitative) dose-response curve?	No (this curve does not represent a *population* of individuals)
Can you obtain the ED_{50} from a quantal (cumulative) dose-response curve?	Yes (this curve represents a *population* of individuals)

What is TD$_{50}$?

Estimation of the toxic dose in 50% of a population; the dose at which 50% of the population will have toxic effects from the drug

What is LD$_{50}$?

Estimation of the lethal dose in 50% of a population; the dose at which 50% of the population will die from the drug

What is therapeutic index (TI)?

The relative safety of a drug by comparing the ED$_{50}$ to either the TD$_{50}$ or LD$_{50}$; the safer the drug, the "wider" the TI, meaning the TD$_{50}$ or LD$_{50}$ is much greater than the ED$_{50}$; drugs with a "narrow" TI have their TD$_{50}$ or LD$_{50}$ close to the ED$_{50}$

How do you calculate TI?

$$TI = \frac{TD_{50}}{ED_{50}} \text{ or } \frac{LD_{50}}{ED_{50}}$$

In the following graph, what is the ED$_{50}$?

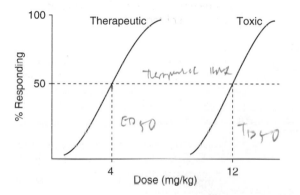

4

In the following graph, what is the TD_{50}?

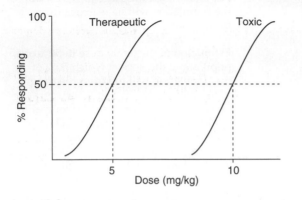

10

In the following graph, what is the TI?

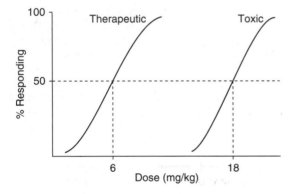

$3; TI = TD_{50}/ED_{50}$
$= 18/6$

What is a narrow therapeutic index (NTI)?

Drugs with an NTI usually have a TI less than 2.

List some examples of drugs with an NTI:

Carbamazepine; digoxin; levothyroxine; lithium; phenytoin; theophylline; valproic acid; warfarin

CLINICAL VIGNETTES

If the ED_{50} of a particular drug is 100 mg and the LD_{50} is 1 g, then what is the drug's therapeutic index (TI)?

TI = 10; TI = LD_{50}/ED_{50}

If 100% of a drug is cleared renally, then what would happen to the drug's half-life if the left kidney was to completely fail?

Increase twofold; $t_{1/2} = (0.7 \times V_d)/(Cl)$; if only one kidney is "working" then the clearance has been cut in half thereby doubling the half-life (half-life is inversely proportional to clearance)

A 57-year-old man, that recently underwent a liver transplant 2 years ago, is currently being immunosuppressed with cyclosporin A. The patient asks his primary care physician if he can take over-the-counter St. John's wort for his "depressed mood." How should the patient's physician respond to this question?

The physician should advise against the use of over-the-counter medications. St. John's wort is an inducer of the cytochrome P-450 enzymes that metabolize cyclosporin A, thereby leading to subtherapeutic serum levels and potentially inducing a graft rejection secondary to inadequate immunosuppression.

A woman who is a long-time Floridian retiree has enjoyed having red grapefruits for breakfast each morning before taking a beach stroll with her friends. Despite her good physical condition she was recently diagnosed with general anxiety disorder and was prescribed triazolam before bedtime. Does the physician need to learn this patient's meal habits before prescribing this medication?

Yes, consumption of fresh grapefruits and grapefruit juice will inhibit the metabolism of triazolam leading to overdosing and increased sedation in an elderly patient.

CHAPTER 2

Antimicrobial Agents

ANTIBACTERIAL AGENTS

What is a bacteriostatic antibiotic?

An antibiotic that causes reversible inhibition of growth. The bacteria are still present and able to replicate should the bacteriostatic antibiotic be removed. A bacteriostatic antibiotic therefore prevents the exponential growth of bacteria, allowing the host immune system better chances of clearing the bacteria that is present in the body.

What is a bactericidal antibiotic?

An antibiotic that causes irreversible inhibition of growth, therefore directly killing the bacteria

Why should bacteriostatic and bactericidal antibiotics not be given together?

Bacteriostatic drugs will antagonize the effects of bacteriocidal drugs which rely on the active replication and utilization of environmental resources by bacteria.

Which antibiotic inhibits bacterial cell wall synthesis by blocking glycopeptide polymerization through binding tightly to the D-alanyl-D-alanine portion of the cell wall (peptidoglycan) precursor?

Vancomycin

Vancomycin-resistant bacteria change their D-ala-D-ala terminus of the peptide side chain to what?

To D-ala-D-lactate; this change prevents the cross linking reaction necessary for elongation of the peptide side chain, weakening the cell wall and making the bacteria susceptible to lysis

Vancomycin is most commonly used to treat what types of infections?

Gram-positive infections. Vancomycin is only effective against gram-positive bacteria, and is particularly useful for infections due to methicillin resistant *Staphylococcus aureus* (MRSA) infections.

Does vancomycin have good oral bioavailability?

metron dnale

No. Vancomycin can be given orally to treat *Clostridium difficile* enterocolitis because the drug stays in the gastrointestinal tract (it is poorly absorbed from the GI tract).

What are the adverse effects of vancomycin?

vanco → red m

Hyperemia, or "red man" syndrome (see following questions); ototoxicity (rare, but it must be used with caution when coadministered with other drugs having ototoxicity, such as aminoglycosides); nephrotoxicity (similar situation as described for ototoxicity); phlebitis at site of injection

Release of what substance is responsible for "red man" syndrome?

VANCO

Histamine

How can vancomycin-induced "red man" syndrome be prevented?

By slowing the infusion rate. Infusion over 1 to 2 hours is normally sufficient. Additionally, antihistamines may be coadministered.

Which antibiotic inhibits the phosphorylation/dephosphorylation cycling of the lipid carrier required in the transfer of peptidoglycan to the cell wall?

Bacitracin (used topically only due to severe nephrotoxicity if given systemically)

Sulfonamide antibiotics antagonize what compound?

Para-aminobenzoic acid (PABA) (see next answer)

What is the mechanism of action of sulfonamide antibiotics?

Sulfonamides are structural analogs of PABA. This class of antibiotics is effective against bacteria that must use PABA to synthesize folate de novo. Sulfonamides work by inhibiting dihydropteroic acid synthase, the enzyme that catalyzes the condensation reaction between PABA and dihydropteridine to form dihydropteroic acid, the first step in the synthesis of tetrahydrofolic acid.

Do humans possess dihydropteroic acid synthase?

No. Therefore sulfonamides are selectively toxic to bacteria and other microorganisms.

Against which microorganisms are sulfonamides effective?

(egn)

Gram-positive and gram-negative bacteria, *Nocardia*, *Chlamydia trachomatis*, some protozoa (malaria), *Escherichia Coli*, *Klebsiella, Salmonella, Shigella, Enterobacter*

nocacha, proleus

Are sulfonamide antibiotics bactericidal or bacteriostatic?

Primarily bacteriostatic (half bacterium ruron)

What are the adverse effects of sulfonamide antibiotics? CN, V, D)

Nausea; vomiting; diarrhea; phototoxicity; hemolysis (in individuals having glucose-6-phosphate dehydrogenase (G6PD) deficiency); hypersensitivity; Stevens-Johnson syndrome (incidence and severity of adverse effects greatly increase immunocompromised in AIDS patients)

Why are sulfonamide antibiotics contraindicated in neonates?

They displace bilirubin from albumin thereby causing kernicterus in neonates.
→ brain dysfnaze

Give examples of sulfonamide antibiotics:

Sulfamethoxazole; sulfacetamide; sulfisoxazole; sulfadiazine (only available in the United States in combination with pyrimethamine); sulfadoxine in combination with pyrimethamine (the antimalarial "Fansidar")

Name antibiotics that works synergistically with sulfonamides by preventing the next reaction in folate synthesis: (Bactrim); TMP-SMX

Trimethoprim or pyrimethamine

What is the mechanism of action of trimethoprim?

Competitive inhibitor of dihydrofolic acid reductase (DHFR), the enzyme that converts dihydrofolic acid to tetrahydrofolic acid

What are the adverse effects of trimethoprim?

Leukopenia; granulocytopenia; thrombocytopenia; megaloblastic anemia

The trimethoprim-sulfamethoxazole combination is most commonly used to treat what type of infections?

Urinary tract infections (UTI) primarily caused by *E. coli* as well as many upper respiratory infections (URI) such as *Pneumocystis jiroveci* pneumonia, some nontuberculous mycobacterial infections, most *S. aureus* strains, *Pneumococcus*, *Haemophilus* sp, *Moraxella catarrhalis*, and *Klebsiella pneumoniae* infections. However, up to 30% of UTI and URI pathogenic strains are resistant to this antibiotic combination.

Give examples of how bacteria may become resistant to sulfonamide antibiotics:

Increased concentrations of PABA; ↑(Paba) decreased binding affinity of target enzymes; uptake and use of exogenous sources of folic acid

What is the mechanism of action of fluoroquinolone antibiotics?

Inhibition of two DNA gyrases (bacterial DNA topoisomerase II and IV) which in turn prevents relaxation of supercoiled DNA inhibiting DNA replication and transcription

Give examples of fluoroquinolone antibiotics:

Ciprofloxacin, moxifloxacin, gemifloxacin, levofloxacin, lomefloxacin, norfloxacin, ofloxacin, gatifloxacin. All are fluorinated derivatives of nalidixic acid giving them the ability to be active systemically.

What types of bacteria are susceptible to quinolone antibiotics?

Many gram-positive and gram-negative bacteria. Examples include *Shigella*, *Salmonella*, toxigenic *E. Coli*, *Campylobacter*, *Pseudomonas*, *Enterobacter*, chlamydial urethritis or cervicitis, and atypical mycobacterial infections

What are the adverse effects of fluoroquinolone antibiotics?

Generally are well tolerated, but nausea, vomiting, and diarrhea are the most common adverse effects. Dizziness, insomnia, headache, photosensitivity, QT interval prolongation also occur with certain quinolones. Gatifloxacin causes hyperglycemia in diabetics and hypoglycemia when used in combination with oral hypoglycemics, and therefore is only available for ophthalmic use in the United States.

Why are fluoroquinolone antibiotics contraindicated in children?

They have deleterious effects on cartilage development, thereby causing tendonitis and possible tendon rupture.

Are fluoroquinolone antibiotics bactericidal or bacteriostatic?

Bactericidal

Give examples of how bacteria may become resistant to fluoroquinolone antibiotics:

Reduced drug penetration (drug efflux pumps); mutations in DNA gyrases result in decreased binding affinity of bacterial target enzymes for fluoroquinolones

What is the mechanism of action of β-lactam antibiotics?

They weaken the cell wall by inactivating transpeptidases (penicillin-binding protein [PBPs]), thereby inhibiting transpeptidation reactions necessary in the cross-linking of peptidoglycan subunits in the bacterial cell wall.

Name the four main classes of β-lactam antibiotics:	1. Penicillins 2. Cephalosporins 3. Carbapenems 4. Monobactams
Give examples of how bacteria may become resistant to β-lactam antibiotics?	Production of β-lactamases (cleaves the β-lactam ring—the most common mechanism); alteration of PBPs; inhibition of drugs to reach PBPs; downregulation of porin structure (only in gram-negative organisms since gram-positive organisms lack the outer cell wall where porins are located); development of efflux pumps in gram-negatives
Which class of β-lactam antibiotics is resistant to β-lactamases?	Monobactams
Give an example of a monobactam antibiotic:	Aztreonam. This is the only monobactam available in the United States.
What organisms are monobactams active against?	Aerobic gram-negative rods, including pseudomonas
Can a monobactam be used in a penicillin-allergic patient?	Yes. This makes monobactams a good choice for patients with a penicillin allergy and a serious gram-negative infection.
Give examples of antibiotics that belong to each of the following penicillin classes:	
β-lactamase susceptible; narrow spectrum	Penicillin G (intravenous); penicillin V (oral)
β-lactamase susceptible; broad spectrum	Amoxicillin; ampicillin; piperacillin; ticarcillin
β-lactamase resistant; narrow spectrum	Methicillin; nafcillin; dicloxacillin; oxacillin
Penicillins are synergistic with what other antibiotic drug class in the treatment of enterococcal and pseudomonal infections?	Aminoglycosides. Aminoglycosides are very polar molecules that cannot easily cross the cell wall. With inhibition of cell wall formation by penicillins, aminoglycosides are then able to enter cells and exert their effects.
Name three β-lactamase inhibitors that can be used in combination with penicillins:	1. Clavulanate 2. Sulbactam 3. Tazobactam

What are the adverse effects of the penicillin antibiotics?

Hypersensitivity; acute interstitial nephritis (common with methicillin); nausea; vomiting; diarrhea; hepatitis (oxacillin); hemolytic anemia; pseudomembranous colitis (ampicillin)

What is the mechanism of methicillin resistance by *S. aureus*?

Production of an alternative PBP 2a

Does *Streptococcus* make β-lactamase?

No (mechanism of resistance is via altered PBPs)

Are β-lactam antibiotics effective in treating *Mycoplasma* infections?

No (*Mycoplasma* have no cell walls)

Give examples of medications in each of the following cephalosporin classes:

Note: It is unnecessary to memorize every drug in each generation. Usually there are two to three cephalosporins on formulary, so their use will vary depending on the particular hospital. Licensing exams will not ask you to choose between cephalosporins in the same generation.

First generation

Cefazolin; cephalexin; cefadroxil; cephapirin; cephradine

Second generation

Cefuroxime; cefotetan; cefaclor; cefoxitin; cefprozil; cefpodoxime; cefamandole; cefmetazole; loracarbef; cefonicid

Third generation

Cefotaxime; Ceftazidime; Ceftriaxone; Cefpodoxime; cefdinir; cefditoren; ceftibuten; cefixime; cefoperazone; ceftizoxime; moxalactam

Fourth generation

Cefepime (only representative drug of this generation)

Which cephalosporin has the broadest spectrum of activity and is resistant to β-lactamases?

Cefepime

How does the antibiotic spectrum of activity of cephalosporins vary by generation, that is, how does the coverage of second-generation drugs compare to first generation and so on?

Second generation: increased gram-negative coverage as compared to first generation. Third generation: continued increase in gram-negative coverage and greater ability to cross blood-brain barrier as compared to second generation drugs. Fourth generation: increased β-lactamase resistance as compared to third-generation drugs

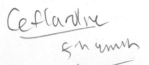

Give examples of carbapenem β- lactams:

Imipenem; meropenem; ertapenem; doripenem

Why is cilastatin given concomitantly with imipenem?

Cilastatin (a dipeptidase inhibitor) inhibits renal dihydropeptidases in the renal tubules which inactivate imipenem, thereby allowing imipenem to exert its effects.

What is the difference in microbial coverage between imipenem and ertapenem?

Ertapenem does not cover *Acinetobacter* species and pseudomonal species.

What is the mechanism of action of aminoglycoside antibiotics?

Binds to 30S ribosomal subunit to prevent formation of initiation complex, thereby inhibiting bacterial protein synthesis; incorporation of incorrect amino acids in the growing peptide chain

Are aminoglycoside antibiotics bactericidal or bacteriostatic?

Bactericidal

Give examples of aminoglycoside antibiotics:

Gentamicin; tobramycin; streptomycin; amikacin; neomycin

What is streptomycin commonly used to treat?

Tuberculosis infections

Why might the efficacy of an aminoglycoside be increased when given as a single large dose as opposed to multiple smaller doses (two reasons)?

1. Concentration-dependent killing: increasing concentrations of aminoglycosides kill a greater proportion of bacteria more quickly.
2. Postantibiotic effect: the antibacterial activity of aminoglycosides lasts longer than detectable levels of the drug are found in the bloodstream.

Against which organisms are aminoglycosides effective?

Gram-negative aerobes. Aminoglycosides passively diffuse across porins in the outer membrane of gram-negatives and their entry across the inner membrane is oxygen dependent. Use with a β-lactam increases gram-positive coverage.

Although synergistic in their clinical effects, why can penicillins and aminoglycosides not be given in the same vial?

The penicillins would directly inactivate the aminoglycosides.

**What are the adverse effects
of the aminoglycoside antibiotics?**

Nephrotoxicity (acute tubular necrosis);
ototoxicity; hypersensitivity;
neuromuscular blockade. Adverse
effects are also dose dependent, just like
efficacy, so close monitoring of drug
levels is necessary. Ototoxicity may be
irreversible; therefore it is imperative to
act before a clinical change in hearing
has occurred.

**In regards to aminoglycoside
ototoxicity, are high-frequency
or low-frequency sounds
affected first?**

High frequency

**Give examples of how bacteria
may become resistant to
aminoglycoside antibiotics?**

Inactivation of drug via conjugation
reactions (acetylation; adenylation;
phosphorylation); inactivation driven
by plasmid-encoded enzymes

**Which aminoglycoside antibiotic
is the most toxic?**

Neomycin (used primarily for topical
application)

**What is the mechanism of
action of clindamycin?**

Binds to 50S ribosomal subunit to
inhibit translocation of peptidyl-tRNA
from acceptor to donor site, thereby
inhibiting bacterial protein synthesis

**Is clindamycin bactericidal
or bacteriostatic?**

Bacteriostatic

**What is the spectrum
of activity of clindamycin?** C G(+)

Gram-positives (eg, penicillin-resistant
Staphylococcus); anaerobes (eg,
Bacteroides sp)

**What major adverse effect
is clindamycin associated with?**

Pseudomembranous colitis
(due to *C. difficile*)

**What is the mechanism
of action of macrolide antibiotics?**

Binds to 50S ribosomal subunit to
inhibit translocation of peptidyl-tRNA
from acceptor to donor site, thereby
inhibiting bacterial protein synthesis

**Give examples of macrolide
antibiotics:**

Erythromycin; clarithromycin;
azithromycin; telithromycin (a ketolide
that is structurally related to the
macrolides)

**Are macrolide antibiotics
bactericidal or bacteriostatic?**

Primarily bacteriostatic

Why is a single dose of azithromycin as effective as a 7-day course of doxycycline for chlamydial infections?

Azithromycin has a very long half-life of 68 hours.

Which of the macrolide (group) antibiotics is relatively free of drug-drug interactions?

Azithromycin

Which macrolide related antibiotic can cause hepatotoxicity and blurred vision?

Telithromycin

What are the clinical uses of telithromycin?

Respiratory tract infections

Give examples of how bacteria may become resistant to macrolide antibiotics:

Alteration of binding sites on the 50S ribosomal subunit; reduced permeability of cell membrane; active efflux; production of esterases by bacteria that hydrolyze the drug

What are the adverse effects of erythromycin? (mainly) GI - m

Nausea; vomiting; diarrhea; anorexia; hepatitis; drug-drug interactions (cytochrome P-450 inhibitor)

What organisms does clarithromycin cover that erythromycin does not?

Mycobacterium avium complex (MAC), *M. leprae, Toxoplasma gondii*

Which macrolide antibiotic is safe in pregnancy?

Azithromycin

What adverse effect is caused by erythromycin given to infants less than 6 weeks of age for pertussis?

Hypertrophic pyloric stenosis

What is the mechanism of action of tetracycline antibiotics?

Binds to 30S ribosomal subunit to inhibit the attachment of aminoacyl-tRNA to its acceptor site, thereby inhibiting bacterial protein synthesis

Give examples of tetracycline antibiotics:

Tetracycline; minocycline; doxycycline; demeclocycline; methacycline

What is demeclocycline used for?

Syndrome of inappropriate antidiuretic hormone (SIADH) via inhibition of antidiuretic hormone (ADH) receptors in the renal collecting ducts

Are tetracycline antibiotics bactericidal or bacteriostatic?

Primarily bacteriostatic

What are the adverse effects of tetracycline antibiotics?	Nausea; vomiting; diarrhea; Fanconi syndrome (outdated tetracyclines); phototoxicity; hepatotoxicity; vestibular toxicity; superinfection
Why are tetracycline antibiotics contraindicated in children?	Tooth enamel dysplasia; permanent discoloration of teeth; decreased bone growth via chelation with calcium salts
Oral absorption of tetracycline antibiotics may be decreased by which multivalent cations?	Iron; calcium; magnesium; aluminum
Give examples of how bacteria may become resistant to tetracycline antibiotics:	Efflux pumps or impaired influx; bacterial production of proteins that decrease binding of tetracyclines to ribosome; enzymatic inactivation
Give an example of a glycylcycline antibiotic (derivative of tetracyclines):	Tigecycline
Is tigecycline effective against MRSA?	Yes
Is tigecycline a substrate for the efflux pump mechanism of resistance to tetracyclines?	No
What is the mechanism of action of chloramphenicol?	Binds to 50S ribosomal subunit to inhibit peptidyltransferase, thereby inhibiting bacterial protein synthesis
What are the adverse effects of chloramphenicol?	Gray baby syndrome in neonates (hypotension, ashen discoloration, vomiting, flaccidity); nausea, vomiting, diarrhea in adults, aplastic anemia; drug-drug interactions (CYP450 inhibitor)
Give examples of streptogramin antibiotics:	Quinupristin; dalfopristin
What is the mechanism of action of streptogramin antibiotics?	Binds 50S ribosomal subunit to inhibit the attachment of aminoacyl-tRNA to its acceptor site, thereby inhibiting bacterial protein synthesis. Specifically, with the fixed dose combination of dalfopristin/quinupristin, dalfopristin distorts the ribosome promoting quinupristin binding. This blocks the aminoacyl-rRNAs from binding to the ribosome and therefore the transpeptidase reaction.

What is the spectrum of action of streptogramin antibiotics?	MRSA; vancomycin-resistant *S. aureus* (VRSA); vancomycin-resistant *Enterococcus faecium* (not *Enterococcus fecalis*)
What are the adverse effects of the streptogramin antibiotics?	Arthralgias; myalgias; drug-drug interactions (CYP450 inhibitor)
Give an example of an oxazolidinone antibiotic:	Linezolid
What is the mechanism of action of linezolid?	Binds to 50S ribosomal subunit to prevent formation of initiation complex, thereby inhibiting bacterial protein synthesis
What are the adverse effects of linezolid?	Nausea; vomiting; diarrhea; headache; bone marrow suppression (primarily thrombocytopenia) after 2 weeks of use; weak reversible inhibitor of (monoamine oxidase) MAO_A and MAO_B; lactic acidosis; peripheral neuropathy; optic neuritis
What is the spectrum of action of linezolid?	Gram-positive organisms such as MRSA; VRSA; vancomycin-resistant *E. faecium* and *E. fecalis*
Give an example of a cyclic lipopeptide antibiotic:	Daptomycin
What is the mechanism of action of daptomycin?	Binds to components of the bacterial cell membrane and causes rapid intracellular depolarization, thereby inhibiting DNA, RNA, and protein synthesis
What is the spectrum of action of daptomycin?	MRSA; VRSA; vancomycin-resistant *E. faecium* and *E. fecalis*, therefore daptomycin is an effective alternative to vancomycin
Which antibiotic, that works by inhibiting protein synthesis, can also be used in patients to increase GI motility?	Erythromycin (activates motilin receptors)

Give the mechanism of action
for each of the following first-line
antituberculosis medications:

Rifampin

Inhibition of DNA-dependent RNA
polymerase

Isoniazid

Inhibition of mycolic acid synthesis

Pyrazinamide

Unknown; activated by susceptible
bacterial strains which in turn
lowers pH of the surrounding
environment

Ethambutol

Inhibition of RNA synthesis

Which of the previous four
antituberculosis medications
is bacteriostatic?

Ethambutol

Give the adverse effects for
each of the following
antituberculosis medications:

Rifampin

Flu-like syndrome; hepatitis; elevated
liver function tests (LFTs); drug-drug
interactions (cytochrome P-450 inducer);
proteinuria; thrombocytopenia; red-
orange discoloration of tears, sweat, urine

Isoniazid

Drug-induced systemic lupus
erythematosus (SLE); hepatitis;
peripheral neuropathy; hemolytic
anemia in G6PD deficiency; seizures

Pyrazinamide

Phototoxicity; increased porphyrin
synthesis; hepatitis; arthralgias;
myalgias; hyperuricemia

Ethambutol

Optic (retrobulbar) neuritis; decreased
visual acuity; red-green color blindness;
hyperuricemia

How can isoniazid-induced
peripheral neuropathy be prevented?

Supplementation of vitamin B_6
(pyridoxine)

ANTIFUNGAL AGENTS

Name two medications
in the polyene antifungal drug class:

Amphotericin B; nystatin

What is the mechanism of action
of the polyene antifungals?

Forms artificial pores by binding to
ergosterol in fungal membranes, thereby
disrupting membrane permeability

How do fungi become resistant to polyene antifungals?

Reduction in the amount of membrane ergosterol

What types of fungi are affected by amphotericin B?

Candida; *Aspergillus*; *Histoplasma*; *Cryptococcus*; *Rhizopus*; *Sporothrix*

Amphotericin B is synergistic with what other antifungal drug in the treatment of candidal and cryptococcal infections?

Flucytosine

+ nucleic acid synthesis

Flucytosine is converted by fungal cytosine deaminase to what active compound?

5-Fluorouracil which is subsequently converted selectively in fungal cells into two other compounds which inhibit DNA and RNA synthesis

Does amphotericin B have good central nervous system (CNS) penetration?

No, amphotericin B must be given via intrathecal route if adequate cerebrospinal fluid (CSF) levels are warranted

Which polyene antifungal is said to cause a "shake and bake" adverse reaction?

IV infusion of amphotericin B can cause fevers, chills, rigors, and hypotension, the so called "shake and bake" adverse reaction.

How can the "shake and bake" adverse reaction caused by amphotericin B be prevented?

Test dose prior to initiation of intravenous therapy; pretreatment with antihistamines, nonsteroidal anti-inflammatory drugs (NSAIDs), meperidine, and glucocorticoids

Pretreatment with meperidine prior to amphotericin B infusion is used to prevent what specific adverse reaction?

Rigors

What is the major dose-limiting adverse effect of amphotericin B?

Nephrotoxicity (also causes anemia via decreased erythropoietin, hypokalemia, hypomagnesemia, decreased glomerular filtration rate [GFR], renal tubular acidosis)

How can the nephrotoxicity caused by amphotericin B be minimized?

Load with normal saline solution; use of amphotericin B in combination with another medication so that the dose of amphotericin B can be decreased; use of liposomal amphotericin B formulations

Give examples of the azole antifungal drug class:

Fluconazole; itraconazole; ketoconazole; voriconazole; miconazole; clotrimazole; posaconazole; ravuconazole

What is the mechanism of action of the azole antifungals?

Prevents the synthesis of ergosterol from lanosterol by inhibiting cytochrome P-450-dependent 14-α-*demethylation*

Fluconazole is the drug of choice for what types of fungal infections?

Mucocutaneous candidiasis; coccidioidomycosis; prevention and treatment of cryptococcal meningitis

Itraconazole is the drug of choice for what types of fungal infections?

Sporotrichoses; blastomycoses

Which antifungal is the drug of choice for paracoccidioides infections?

Ketoconazole

What antifungal can be formulated into a topical shampoo gel to treat dermatophytosis of the scalp?

Ketoconazole

What is another name for dermatophytosis of the scalp?

Tinea capitis

What adverse effect of ketoconazole is also an adverse effect of spironolactone?

Gynecomastia (via inhibition of androgen synthesis)

Voriconazole can be used to treat what types of fungal infections?

Invasive aspergillosis; invasive candidiasis; candidemia

Is absorption of ketoconazole increased or decreased by alkalinization of gastric pH?

It is decreased. Do not use antacids in combination with ketoconazole.

Some physicians may tell patients to drink what in order to enhance the oral absorption of ketoconazole?

Coca-Cola, Pepsi-Cola, etc. Carbonated beverages that contain phosphoric and/or citric acid are acidic and therefore enhance oral absorption.

The International Normalized Ratio (INR) of a patient stabilized on warfarin therapy will be increased or decreased when an azole antifungal medication is initiated?

Increased (azole antifungals inhibit hepatic cytochrome P-450 enzymes thereby inhibiting the metabolism and increasing the blood levels of warfarin)

Which laboratory tests may become elevated in patients being treated with azole antifungals?

Liver function tests (LFTs) used to monitor for hepatotoxicity

Which antifungal medications act by inhibiting the synthesis of β-(1-3)-d-glucan?

Caspofungin; anidulafungin; micafungin

↓ echinocandins cell walls

β-(1-3)-d-Glucan is an integral part of the fungal cell membrane or fungal cell wall?

Fungal cell wall

Caspofungin can be used to treat what types of fungal infections?

Invasive aspergillosis; invasive candidiasis; candidemia

Which antifungal, active only against dermatophytes, acts by depositing in newly formed keratin and disrupting microtubule structure?

Griseofulvin

↓MT for derm

Griseofulvin is active against dermatophytes when used orally or topically?

When used orally

What is the major dose-limiting adverse reaction of griseofulvin?

Hepatotoxicity

Griseofulvin is contraindicated in patients with which disease?

Acute intermittent porphyria

Name the three major dermatophytes:

1. Epidermophyton
2. Trichophyton
3. Microsporum

Which antifungal inhibits ergosterol synthesis by inhibiting squalene epoxidase?

Terbinafine

Terbinafine is used to treat what types of fungal infections?

Dermatophytic infections

Oral terbinafine is used to treat what specific types of dermatophytic infections?

Onychomycosis of the toenail; onychomycosis of the fingernail

Oral terbinafine can cause what major dose-limiting adverse reaction?

Hepatotoxicity

ANTIVIRAL AGENTS

What enzyme adds the first phosphate to acyclovir?

Viral thymidine kinase

True or False? Monophosphorylated acyclovir is converted to the triphosphate form by viral enzymes.

False (host cell kinases are responsible for these reactions)

How does acyclovir triphosphate work as an antiviral agent?

Inhibits viral DNA replication by competing with deoxyguanosine triphosphate for viral DNA polymerase; incorporated into the viral DNA molecule and acts as a chain terminator

How does acyclovir triphosphate work as a chain terminator?

Lacks the ribosyl 3′ hydroxyl group

How do viruses become resistant to acyclovir?

Downregulation of viral thymidine kinase; lacking thymidine kinase altogether; altered specificity of viral thymidine kinase; altered specificity of viral DNA polymerase

Acyclovir is effective in treating which virus types?

Herpes simplex virus (HSV) 1 and 2; varicella-zoster virus (VZV). Acyclovir is 10 × more potent against HSV than VZV.

Is acyclovir effective in treating postherpetic neuralgia?

No (only effective against acute neuritis)

What is the oral bioavailability of acyclovir?

15%-30%. There is minimal systemic distribution after topical application.

What is the half-life of acyclovir in adults?

2.5-3 hours

Why is it necessary to maintain adequate hydration in patients receiving IV acyclovir therapy?

To prevent crystalluria or interstitial nephritis. Slow infusion additionally helps to avoid these adverse reactions.

What is the name of the prodrug that is converted to acyclovir and L-valine by first-pass metabolism?

Valacyclovir

What is the advantage of valacyclovir over acyclovir?

Higher oral bioavailability of 54%-70%

Famciclovir is a prodrug that is metabolized to what active metabolite?

Penciclovir

What is the bioavailability of penciclovir after oral administration of famciclovir?

70%

Is famciclovir effective in viral strains resistant to acyclovir secondary to mutated DNA polymerase?

Yes

Is famciclovir effective in viral strains resistant to acyclovir secondary to lack of thymidine kinase?

No

What is the mechanism of action of ganciclovir?

Phosphorylated to a substrate which competitively inhibits binding of deoxyguanosine triphosphate to DNA polymerase, thereby inhibiting viral DNA synthesis

Does ganciclovir have chain-terminating ability?

No

Ganciclovir is effective in treating which virus types?

HSV; VZV; human herpes virus (HHV)-6 and 8; cytomegalovirus (CMV). Activity against CMV is 100× greater than acyclovir. It may be used intraocularly for CMV retinitis.

What is the advantage of valganciclovir over its parent drug ganciclovir?

Valganciclovir (the valine ester) has up to 60% better oral availability than ganciclovir.

What is ganciclovir's dose-limiting adverse effect?

Myelosuppression; thrombocytopenia; anemia; leukopenia

What are the adverse effects of ganciclovir?

Crystalluria; mucositis; rash; fever; hepatotoxicity; seizures; diarrhea; nausea; hematotoxicity

What is cidofovir used for?

CMV retinitis most commonly. It also has activity against HSV-1 and 2, varicella zoster virus (VZV), Epstein-Barr virus (EBV), HHV-6 and 8, adenovirus, poxviruses, polyomaviruses, and human papilloma virus (HPV).

What antiviral agent is a pyrophosphate analogue that acts as an inhibitor of viral RNA and DNA polymerase and HIV reverse transcriptase?

Foscarnet

Does foscarnet require activation by thymidine kinase?

No

Foscarnet is effective in treating which virus types?

Acyclovir-resistant HSV and VZV; ganciclovir-resistant CMV

Does foscarnet cause hematotoxicity?

Yes

What are the major adverse effects of foscarnet?

Hematotoxicity; fever; seizures; electrolyte abnormalities; nausea; vomiting; diarrhea

What types of electrolyte abnormalities can foscarnet cause?

Hyper- or hypocalcemia; hyper- or hypomagnesemia; hyper- or hypophosphatemia; hypokalemia

True of False? Amantadine is effective in treating both influenza A and B.

False (it is effective against the influenza A virus only)

What is the antiviral mechanism of action of amantadine?

Blocks the uncoating of influenza A virus, thereby preventing penetration of the virus into host cells

What other noninfectious disease processes is amantadine used for?

Parkinson disease; drug-induced extrapyramidal symptoms. It also increases dopamine levels in the synaptic cleft by either inhibiting reuptake into presynaptic neurons or by increasing release from presynaptic neurons. It may have anticholinergic effects.

What are the adverse effects of amantadine?

Seizures; insomnia; nervousness; livedo reticularis; orthostatic hypotension; peripheral edema; dry nose; xerostomia; nausea; anorexia

What is livedo reticularis?

A purplish discoloration of the skin caused by dilation of capillaries and venules secondary to stasis or changes in underlying blood vessels

Name two drugs that inhibit neuraminidase of both influenza A and B, thereby decreasing the likelihood of viral penetration into host cells:	Oseltamivir; zanamivir
Which neuraminidase inhibitor has an oral inhalational route of administration?	Zanamivir
Ribavirin is effective in treating which virus types?	Respiratory syncytial virus (RSV); influenza A and B; hepatitis C virus (HCV)
Ribavirin is used in conjunction with what other drug to treat HCV?	Interferon-alpha (IFN-α)
What are the adverse effects of ribavirin?	Anemia; neutropenia; thrombocytopenia; anorexia; headache; conjunctivitis; nausea; pharyngitis; lacrimation; alopecia; rash; flu-like syndrome; teratogenicity (pregnancy category X)
Name the major adverse effects of IFN-α:	Flu-like symptoms; depression; alopecia; insomnia; nausea
What is the name of the only available nucleotide reverse transcriptase inhibitor?	Tenofovir
Give examples of nucleoside reverse transcriptase inhibitors (NRTIs):	Zidovudine (AZT); stavudine (d4T); lamivudine (3TC); didanosine (ddI); abacavir (ABC); emtricitabine (FTC)
What adverse effect(s) are associated with all NRTIs?	Lactic acidosis with hepatic steatosis
What is the general mechanism of action of NRTIs?	Interference with HIV viral RNA-dependent DNA polymerase resulting in inhibition of HIV viral replication
What two NRTIs are thymidine analogs?	Zidovudine; stavudine
What NRTI is an adenosine analog?	Didanosine
What NRTI is a guanosine analog?	Abacavir

What two NRTIs are cytosine analogs?	1. Emtricitabine 2. Lamivudine
Which NRTI should not be rechallenged if hypersensitivity is expected?	Abacavir (symptoms include fever, rash, nausea, vomiting, malaise, fatigue, and respiratory dysfunction)
Which NRTI can cause hyperuricemia?	Didanosine
Which two NRTIs can cause pancreatitis?	1. Didanosine 2. Stavudine (dose-limiting effect)
Which two NRTIs can cause peripheral neuropathy?	1. Didanosine 2. Stavudine (dose-limiting effect)
What is didanosine's dose-limiting adverse effect?	Pancreatitis
What is stavudine's dose-limiting adverse effect?	Peripheral neuropathy
What are the main adverse effects of AZT?	Anemia and neutropenia (dose-limiting effect/potentiated by vitamin B_{12}); headache; nausea; insomnia; body aches; lactic acidosis
What is the dose-limiting adverse effect of AZT?	Hematotoxicity
What antiretroviral agent can cause Fanconi syndrome?	Tenofovir. Fanconi syndrome is impairment of the proximal tubule resulting in increased phosphate and calcium losses.
What NRTI can cause altered LFTs, lipoatrophy, hyperlipidemia, and ascending paresis?	Stavudine
Name three nonnucleoside reverse transcriptase inhibitors (NNRTIs):	1. Delavirdine 2. Efavirenz 3. Nevirapine
What is the mechanism of action of efavirenz?	Binds directly to reverse transcriptase and blocks the RNA-and DNA-dependent DNA polymerase activity of reverse transcriptase
What is the class adverse effect(s) of the NNRTIs?	Rash
Which NNRTI can cause hepatitis and hepatic necrosis?	Nevirapine

Which NNRTI can cause abnormal dreams, impaired concentration, dizziness, and altered LFTs?	Efavirenz
Which NNRT can produce a false-positive urine test for Cannabis?	Efavirenz (in about 50% of patients)
Do NNRTIs require metabolic activation?	No
Do NRTIs require metabolic activation?	Yes
What is the name of the drug that inhibits fusion of the HIV-1 virus with CD4 cells by binding to and blocking the conformational change in gp41 required for membrane fusion and entry into CD4 cells?	Enfuvirtide (fusion inhibitor)
What are the adverse effects of enfuvirtide?	Pain, induration, erythema, and nodules at the injection site; nausea; vomiting; diarrhea; fatigue
Give examples of protease inhibitors:	Atazanavir; indinavir; lopinavir; fosamprenavir; nelfinavir; ritonavir; saquinavir; tipranavir; amprenavir; darunavir
What adverse effect(s) are associated with the protease inhibitors?	Hepatotoxicity; fat maldistribution; insulin resistance; osteonecrosis; increased bleeding in hemophiliac patients
Are protease inhibitors metabolized by P-450 enzymes?	Yes
Do protease inhibitors inhibit or induce P-450 enzymes?	They inhibit P-450 enzymes.
What is HIV protease responsible for?	Cleaves the Gag-Pol polyprotein of HIV (the gag region of the gene codes for structural proteins whereas the Pol region of the gene codes for protease, reverse transcriptase, and integrase)
The combination of atazanavir and indinavir can cause what possible adverse effect?	Hyperbilirubinemia

Patients with sulfonamide allergy should use caution when taking which two protease inhibitors?	1. Tipranavir 2. Fosamprenavir
Which protease inhibitor can cause an altered taste sensation?	Ritonavir
Which two protease inhibitors can cause asthenia (lack of strength)?	1. Lopinavir 2. Ritonavir
Which protease inhibitor can cause kidney stone formation?	Indinavir
Which protease inhibitor can cause numbness around the mouth?	Ritonavir
What type of prophylaxis is given to a person stuck with a potentially HIV contaminated needle?	Zidovudine and lamivudine for 1 month (protease inhibitor should be added for high-risk exposures)
How is maternal-fetal HIV transmission prevented in mothers?	Zidovudine beginning at 14-34 weeks' gestation and continued until start of labor; during labor and delivery, zidovudine until the umbilical cord is clamped
How is maternal-fetal HIV transmission prevented in neonates?	Zidovudine started 8-12 hours after birth and continued for 6 weeks

ANTIPROTOZOAL AGENTS

Amebiasis is generally treated with what drug combination?	Metronidazole and diloxanide
What is the mechanism of action of metronidazole?	Mixed amebicide (effective against both luminal and systemic forms of disease); nitro group of metronidazole acts as an electron acceptor, thereby forming reduced cytotoxic compounds that lead to inhibition of protein synthesis and DNA strand breakage
What are the adverse effects of metronidazole?	Nausea; vomiting; metallic taste sensation; disulfiram-like reaction
Give examples of medications that can cause a disulfiram-like reaction:	Metronidazole; chlorpropamide; cefotetan; cefamandole; cefoperazone

What is the antimicrobial spectrum of metronidazole?	*Entamoeba histolytica; Giardia lamblia; Trichomonas vaginalis;* bacterial anaerobes; *C. difficile*
Metronidazole is contraindicated in which trimester of pregnancy?	First trimester during organogenesis since teratogenicity has not been effectively ruled out
Can metronidazole cross the blood-brain barrier (BBB)?	Yes
What is the mechanism of action of diloxanide?	Luminal amebicide (effective against luminal forms of disease) used in the treatment of asymptomatic amoebic cyst passers
What are the adverse effects of diloxanide?	Contraindicated in pregnancy and children less than 2 years old; dry mouth; pruritus; flatulence
What are the four species of *Plasmodium*?	1. *Malariae* 2. *Falciparum* 3. *Vivax* 4. *Ovale*
What is the most dangerous/ life-threatening *Plasmodium* species?	*Falciparum*
What are the three stages of the malarial parasite life cycle primarily targeted by antimalarial drugs?	1. Erythrocytic stage 2. Exoerythrocytic stage 3. Gametocytic stage
What is the oldest antimalarial drug still in use?	Quinine ("Jesuit Bark")
Quinine has been replaced by which antimalarial drug?	Chloroquine (more potent and less toxic than quinine)
What drugs are effective against the exoerythrocytic forms of malaria?	Primaquine; atovaquone + proguanil (Malarone)
What drug is effective against the gametocytic (hepatic) forms of malaria?	Primaquine
Is primaquine effective against erythrocytic forms of malaria?	No
Give examples of antimalarial drugs that are effective against the erythrocytic forms of malaria:	Hydroxychloroquine; chloroquine; mefloquine; pyrimethamine; quinine; atovaquone + proguanil; artemisinin

What drug is effective against relapsing forms of *P. vivax* and *P. ovale* malarias?

Primaquine. To prevent recurrence of infection, hepatic forms of these parasites must be eliminated.

What are the adverse effects of primaquine?

Hemolytic anemia in patients with G6PD deficiency; methemoglobinemia; agranulocytosis

What is the drug of choice for acute attacks of malaria caused by chloroquine-sensitive strains of *P. falciparum* and *P. vivax*?

Chloroquine

Does chloroquine have a large or small V_d?

Large

What is the mechanism of action of chloroquine?

It concentrates within parasite food vacuoles and raises pH leading to inhibition of growth; inhibits hemoglobin metabolism and utilization by parasites; concentrates within parasite vacuoles and raises pH leading to inhibition of growth; binds to ferriprotoporphyrin IX leading to membrane damage; inhibits DNA and RNA polymerase

What continents contain the largest repositories of chloroquine-resistant *P. falciparum*?

Africa, Asia

What are the adverse effects of chloroquine?

ECG changes (quinidine-like effects); headaches; pruritus; mucosal pigmentary changes (blue-black); photosensitivity; nausea; vomiting; diarrhea; aplastic anemia; agranulocytosis; neutropenia; thrombocytopenia; retinopathy; tinnitus; reduced hearing

Chloroquine is contraindicated in patients with what disease states?

Porphyria; psoriasis

What are the major adverse effects of quinine?

Cinchonism (nausea, vomiting, diarrhea, tinnitus, vertigo); hemolytic anemia; digoxin toxicity

What other medication can cause cinchonism?

Quinidine

Is quinine acidic or basic?	Basic
How can the urinary excretion of quinine (or chloroquine) be enhanced?	Acidification of the urine
Name two newer antimalarials that are chemically related to quinine:	1. Halofantrine 2. Lumefantrine
What can be used to acidify the urine?	Ammonium chloride
What is the mechanism of action of pyrimethamine?	Inhibits nucleic acid and protein metabolism in the parasites; plasmodial dihydrofolate reductase (DHFR) inhibitor
The antimalarial effects of pyrimethamine can be potentiated by combining it with which drugs?	Sulfonamides (synergistic blockade of folic acid synthesis).
How is folate-deficient megaloblastic anemia reversed in patients taking pyrimethamine?	Leucovorin
What is the mechanism of action of leucovorin?	As a reduced form of folic acid, leucovorin supplies human cells with the necessary cofactor blocked by DHFR inhibitors.
What kind of compounds are the antimalarial drug artemisinin and its derivatives?	Sesquiterpene lactones (the active ingredient in a 2000-year-old Chinese herb—Qing Hao).
What is the antimalarial mechanism of action of artemisinin?	It is thought that it is activated by heme to irreversibly decompose generating free radicals that form adducts mostly with proteins and lipids.
Give examples of antimalarial drugs used in artemisinin combination therapies (ACT):	Pyrimethamine/sulfadoxine (Fansidar), mefloquine, amodiaquine
What is the name of the most promising antimalarial vaccine?	RTS-S/AS02A or Mosquirix
Which genetic diseases/ conditions may help protect against malarial infections?	Sickle cell trait; G6PD deficiency

Trypanosoma cruzi is responsible for causing what disease?

American trypanosomiasis (Chagas disease)

T. brucei gambiense and *T. brucei rhodesiense* are responsible for causing what disease?

African trypanosomiasis (sleeping sickness)

What drug is used as a suppressive agent in patients with acute *T. cruzi* infections?

Nifurtimox

What is the mechanism of action of nifurtimox?

Forms intracellular oxygen-free radicals which are toxic to the parasite because of its lack of catalase (oxygen radical scavenger)

What drug is used to treat African sleeping sickness with CNS involvement?

Eflornithine for West African trypanosomiasis; melarsoprol for East African trypanosomiasis

What are the adverse events of melarsoprol?

Hypersensitivity; abdominal pain; vomiting; hemolytic anemia in patients with G6PD deficiency; encephalopathy

What two drugs are used in the early stages of African sleeping sickness?

1. Pentamidine (first choice for West African sleeping sickness)
2. Suramin (first choice for East African sleeping sickness)

Does pentamidine cross the BBB?

No. Therefore it cannot be used for late trypanosomiasis with CNS involvement.

What are the two routes of administration of pentamidine?

1. IV
2. Aerosol

What fungus is pentamidine commonly used to treat?

Pneumocystis carinii

What drug combination is used for prophylaxis against *P. carinii*?

Trimethoprim-sulfamethoxazole

What is the treatment of choice for *T. gondii*?

Pyrimethamine + sulfadiazine

How do humans become infected with *T. gondii*?

Ingestion of undercooked, infected meat; contact with infected cats

Can pregnant mothers transmit *T. gondii* to the fetus?	Yes (remember TORCH syndromes)
What are the three types of leishmaniasis infections?	1. Visceral 2. Cutaneous 3. Mucocutaneous
What is the drug of choice for treating leishmaniasis?	Stibogluconate (pentavalent antimony compound)

ANTIHELMINTHIC AGENTS

What is another name for the nematodes?	Roundworms
What is another name for the trematodes?	Flukes
What is another name for the cestodes?	Tapeworms
What drug is commonly used to treat trematode infections?	Praziquantel
What is the mechanism of action of praziquantel?	Increases cell permeability to calcium, thereby increasing contractions with subsequent paralysis of musculature
What is the mechanism of action of mebendazole?	It irreversibly blocks glucose uptake; inhibits microtubule polymerization
What are the adverse effects of mebendazole?	Diarrhea; abdominal pain; contraindicated during pregnancy
What is the mechanism of action of albendazole?	It interferes with microtubule polymerization; inhibits adenosine triphosphate (ATP) production thereby depleting energy availability
What is the mechanism of action of thiabendazole?	Inhibits helminth-specific mitochondrial fumarate reductase
What types of cutaneous adverse effects are caused by thiabendazole?	Stevens-Johnson syndrome; erythema multiforme

What is the mechanism of action of pyrantel?

Depolarizing neuromuscular blocker thereby causing paralysis of musculature

What types of helminths are affected by praziquantel?

Trematodes; cestodes

What types of helminths are affected by mebendazole?

Nematodes

What types of helminths are affected by pyrantel?

Nematodes

What is the drug of choice for treating *Enterobius vermicularis*?

Mebendazole

What is the common name for *E. vermicularis*?

Pinworm

What is the drug of choice for treating *Onchocerca volvulus* (onchocerciasis or river blindness)?

Ivermectin

What is the mechanism of action of ivermectin?

Acts at helminthic gamma-aminobutyric acid (GABA) receptors, thereby enhancing influx of chloride and causing hyperpolarization and paralysis

Why does onchocerciasis potentially lead to blindness?

A bacteria (*Wolbachia* sp.) that colonizes many parasitic worms, including the nematode that causes onchocerciasis, is an important factor in the inflammatory response that leads to blindness.

What is another name for onchocerciasis?

River blindness

What drug is commonly used to treat cestode infections?

Niclosamide

What is the mechanism of action of niclosamide?

Inhibits mitochondrial phosphorylation of ADP to ATP, thereby depleting energy availability

Is niclosamide active against the ova of cestodes?

No; only active against cestode's scolex and segments

CLINICAL VIGNETTES

A 48-year-old female marine animal trainer develops a reddish granuloma on her hand. Her past medical history is significant only for gastroesophageal reflux disease (GERD) which is well controlled with a PPI (omeprazole). Moreover, she is very conscious as to maintain fitness in keeping with her required scuba licensing; thus, she regularly takes calcium tablets with her meals. She is diagnosed with a *Mycobacterium marinum* infection and begins treatment with minocycline. However, 6 weeks after treatment her condition has not resolved and she has developed new granulomas. What is the most likely reason for treatment failure in this patient?

This vignette underscores the importance of taking a good patient's history. Here the patient's occupation, gender, age, fitness requirements, and medication history are crucial. Her unique occupation gives the patient exposure to microorganisms that are uncommonly causes of infection in the lay human population. In terms of her medications, even supplements have significant side effects and drug interactions, and must be asked about as part of your history. Calcium salts such as those used to increase calcium intake in menopausal women will chelate tetracyclines like minocycline, decreasing their oral bioavailability. Therefore, this patient should have been instructed not to take her calcium supplement tablets 2 hours before or after a dose of her antibiotic.

A 76-year-old man is brought to the intensive care unit (ICU) after being found unresponsive on the floor of his home. It is unknown how long the patient had remained immobile on the floor. Respiratory effort was diminished and the patient was intubated and placed on a ventilator. The intern on call placed the patient on a tobramycin nebulizer to suppress ventilator-associated pneumonia. The next morning, the attending physician sees this and immediately terminates this treatment. Why is tobramycin contraindicated in this patient?

Prolonged immobility leads to dehydration and muscle breakdown with release of creatine phosphokinase (CPK), both of which can cause acute renal failure. Aminoglycosides, such as tobramycin, are nephrotoxic and will cause further damage to the kidneys. All aminoglycosides should be used with caution in the elderly. Another consideration is ototoxicity. Since this patient is unresponsive, we are unaware of his baseline hearing status. A small amount of damage in an individual who is already hard of hearing could have dramatic consequences.

A 24-year-old female medical student participates in an exchange program in rural South Korea. Despite chemoprophylaxis (mefloquine), she develops cyclic shaking chills and fever and is diagnosed with malaria. Treatment is begun with chloroquine, but the student fails to respond. Resistance to chloroquine is suspected, and the treatment is switched to quinidine plus a tetracycline with complete resolution of her symptoms. Two months after her return to the United States, she has a reoccurrence of the malarial symptom⌐   ⌐s this therapy failed to resolve her illness?

The student has most likely contracted *P. vivax*, an end⌐   ⌐laria on the Korean peninsula. Chloroquine (and mefloquine) re   ⌐ncreasing problem worldwide. A quinidine plus tetracycline (eg, d   ⌐ombination is an effective treatment regimen for eradication of chloroquine-resistant malaria. However, it is important to remember that *P. vivax* has liver repositories which the above antimalarial will not treat effectively. Reactivation of these hypnozoites can lead to recurrence of infection months to years later. Once the original acute attack *P. vivax* malaria is resolved, primaquine is the drug of choice to eradicate the liver forms and must be added to the drug regimen in cases of *P. vivax* or *P. ovale*.

Note: Licensing exams will not expect you to determine whether a specific geographic area is endemic with chloroquine resistant strains of malaria. You should know treatment alternatives for drug-resistant strains, as well as when addition of primaquine is necessary to eradicate hepatic repositories of the malaria parasite (ie, therapy is specie-specific).

During the second week of a trip to Belize, a traveler experienced some diarrhea, which was sufficient to remind him of previous admonitions about consuming food dispensed by street vendors. Fortunately, his symptoms seem to subside and he recovered in a few days. About a month after his return, the traveler developed severe pain in the right upper quadrant of his abdomen. When the abdominal pain persisted, he went to a gastroenterologist. The gastroenterologist performed an x-ray study of the intestine after a barium enema, a CT scan, and a serological test for *E. histolytica*. The results of these tests revealed pseudopolyps consistent with inflammatory bowel disease, the CT scan showed abscesses in the liver and a hemagglutination titer of 1:2000 for *E. histolytica*. What antiprotozoal drug should be given to this patient?

The drug of choice for this active amebic infection picture is metronidazole. It is absorbed rapidly from oral doses with a half-life in serum of about 8 hours. It has potent activity against *E. histolytica*. The drug is well tolerated and adverse effects are not common, but nausea, headaches, and dry mouth can occur.

CHAPTER 3

Cancer Chemotherapeutic Agents

BASIC PHARMACOLOGY OF CANCER CHEMOTHERAPEUTICS

According to the log-kill hypothesis, does the cytotoxic action of anticancer drugs follow first-order or second-order kinetics?

First-order kinetics

With first-order kinetics, is it a fixed amount or fixed percentage of tumor cells that are killed by cancer chemotherapeutic agents?

Fixed percentage

If a chemotherapy treatment leads to a 4 log-kill reduction, then how many tumor cells would remain if there were 10^{10} tumor cells to begin with?

10^6 (or $10^{10}/10^4$)

Give a brief summary of what happens during each of the following phases of the cell cycle:

G_0

Cells are not actively dividing (resting state).

G_1

Enzymes and proteins required for DNA replication are synthesized.

S

Replication of DNA

G_2

Enzymes and proteins required for mitosis are synthesized.

M

Mitosis occurs.

The ratio of proliferating (malignant) cells to nonproliferating (G_0) cells is also known as what?	Growth fraction
Are tumor cells more susceptible to cancer chemotherapeutic agents when they are actively dividing or when they are dormant?	Actively dividing. Thus, tumor cells which are dormant may not be sufficiently susceptible to the effects of cancer chemotherapeutic agents.
What is the definition of a cell-cycle specific (CCS) cancer chemotherapeutic agent?	An agent that kills actively dividing cells (cells currently going through the cell cycle)
Give examples of normal/ nonmalignant cells in the body that normally are undergoing rapid proliferation:	Bone marrow cells; GI mucosal cells; hair cells. Thus, the common side effects of chemotherapy include myelosuppression, GI disturbances, and alopecia.
P-glycoprotein is an ATP-dependent membrane (efflux) transporter that is responsible for what?	Pumping drugs out of cells (responsible for multidrug resistance of chemotherapeutic agents)

Give examples of cancer chemotherapeutic agents that are commonly associated with each of the following adverse effects:

Cardiotoxicity; dilated cardiomyopathy	Doxorubicin
Pulmonary fibrosis; pneumonitis	Bleomycin
Stomatitis; esophagitis	Methotrexate; 5-fluorouracil; dactinomycin
Hemorrhagic cystitis	Cyclophosphamide; ifosfamide
Hemorrhagic diathesis	Plicamycin
Peripheral neuropathy; neurotoxicity	Vincristine
Nephrotoxicity	Cisplatin
Allergic reactions	Etoposide; L-asparaginase
Hepatotoxicity	6-Mercaptopurine; busulfan; cyclophosphamide
Pancreatitis	L-Asparaginase
Cutaneous toxicity (hand-foot syndrome)	5-Fluorouracil
Disulfiram-type reactions	Procarbazine

What is the name of the antidote that binds to and inactivates the toxic metabolites responsible for cisplatin-induced nephrotoxicity?	Amifostine
What is the name of the cyclophosphamide and ifosfamide urotoxic metabolite that is responsible for causing hemorrhagic cystitis?	Acrolein
What is the name of the antidote that binds to and inactivates acrolein, thereby preventing hemorrhagic cystitis in patients receiving cyclophosphamide or ifosfamide chemotherapy?	Mesna
Which iron chelating agent is used to decrease the incidence and severity of doxorubicin-induced cardiomyopathy in patients with metastatic breast cancer who have received a lifetime cumulative doxorubicin dose (300 mg/m^2)?	Dexrazoxane
Give examples of antimetabolite cancer chemotherapeutic agents:	Methotrexate; 5-fluorouracil; cytarabine; fludarabine; 6-thioguanine; 6-mercaptopurine
Are the antimetabolite cancer chemotherapeutic agents CCS?	Yes (S phase)
What is the mechanism of action of methotrexate?	Inhibits dihydrofolate reductase (DHFR)
What reaction does DHFR catalyze?	Conversion of folic acid to tetrahydrofolic acid (active form)
What drug is used as a "rescue medication" in patients taking methotrexate?	Leucovorin, which acts as an active form of folic acid (replenishing the folate pool) that has bypassed the inhibited DHFR and is more readily taken up by normal cells than by malignant cells
What are the adverse effects of methotrexate?	Stomatitis; bone marrow suppression (BMS); urticaria; alopecia; nausea; vomiting; diarrhea; nephrotoxicity; hepatotoxicity; pulmonary toxicity; neurotoxicity

What is the mechanism of action of 5-fluorouracil?	Pyrimidine analog that is converted to active 5-FdUMP which inhibits thymidylate synthetase, thereby decreasing the amount of cellular thymidine and subsequent DNA
What is the mechanism of action of cytarabine?	Pyrimidine antagonist
What is the mechanism of action of both 6-mercaptopurine and 6-thioguanine?	Purine antagonists
What immunosuppressive drug becomes active only after being converted to 6-mercaptopurine?	Azathioprine
Because 6-mercaptopurine is metabolized by xanthine oxidase, its serum levels may be significantly increased when given concomitantly with what other medication?	Allopurinol (xanthine oxidase inhibitor)
What enzyme activates 6-mercaptopurine to its corresponding nucleotide form by adding a ribose phosphate to its structure?	Hypoxanthine-guanine phosphoribosyl transferase (HGPRT)
What are the major adverse effects of 6-mercaptopurine?	Nausea; vomiting; diarrhea; hepatotoxicity; BMS
Give examples of antitumor antibiotics:	Doxorubicin; daunorubicin; dactinomycin; plicamycin; bleomycin; idarubicin
Are the antitumor antibiotics CCS?	Yes (S-phase)
Name three anthracycline antitumor antibiotics:	1. Doxorubicin 2. Daunorubicin 3. Idarubicin
What is the mechanism of action of the anthracycline antibiotics?	Inhibition of DNA topoisomerase II; formation of free radicals (leading to DNA strand scission); DNA intercalation; inhibition of DNA and RNA synthesis
Name three non-anthracycline antitumor antibiotics:	1. Dactinomycin 2. Bleomycin 3. Mitomycin

What is the mechanism of action of bleomycin?	Complexes with iron and reacts with oxygen which in turn leads to DNA strand scission
Which phase of the cell cycle is bleomycin specific for?	G_2
Give examples of anticancer alkylating agents:	Cyclophosphamide; ifosfamide; mechlorethamine; nitrosoureas (carmustine, lomustine, streptozotocin); cisplatin; carboplatin
Are the anticancer alkylating chemotherapeutic agents CCS?	No
What is the mechanism of action of anticancer alkylating agents?	Covalently bind (alkylation) to DNA leading to cross-linked and dysfunctional DNA strands
Give examples of anticancer mitotic inhibitors:	Paclitaxel; docetaxel; vincristine; vinblastine; vinorelbine
Are the anticancer mitotic inhibitors CCS?	Yes (M phase)
What is the mechanism of action of vincristine and vinblastine?	They are vinca alkaloids that inhibits the ability of tubulin to polymerize, thereby preventing formation of the microtubule structures needed during mitosis.
What adverse effects do vincristine and vinblastine have in common?	Nausea; vomiting; diarrhea; alopecia; phlebitis; cellulites
Are vincristine and vinblastine vesicants?	Yes, they are strong vesicants.
Which adverse effect is unique to vincristine?	Peripheral neuropathy
Which adverse effect is unique to vinblastine?	BMS
What plant are the vinca alkaloids derived from?	Periwinkle plant
Which plant is paclitaxel a derivative of?	Needles of the Western or Pacific yew tree

What is the mechanism of action of paclitaxel?	Binds to tubulin and increases polymerization and stabilization of the microtubule structure, thereby preventing depolymerization
What are the adverse effects of paclitaxel?	Neutropenia; alopecia; hypersensitivity reactions
How are hypersensitivity reactions prevented in patients receiving paclitaxel cancer chemotherapy?	Pretreatment with diphenhydramine and dexamethasone
Give two examples of epipodophyllotoxin cancer chemotherapeutic agents:	1. Etoposide 2. Teniposide
What is the mechanism of action of the epipodophyllotoxin cancer chemotherapeutic agents?	Inhibition of DNA topoisomerase II
Give two examples of cancer chemotherapeutic agents that inhibit DNA topoisomerase I:	1. Topotecan 2. Irinotecan
What is the mechanism of action of L-asparaginase?	Hydrolyzes asparagine to aspartic acid and ammonia, thereby depriving tumor cells of asparagine required for protein synthesis

This short chapter is meant as an overview of basic concepts of cancer chemotherapy. Clinical pharmacological therapies for specific cancer subtypes are discussed later in the text in relevant chapters.

CHAPTER 4

Autonomic Agents

CHOLINERGIC AGENTS

What are the major subdivisions of the autonomic nervous system?

It is divided into the sympathetic and the parasympathetic nervous systems.

What is the major neurotransmitter of the parasympathetic autonomic nervous system?

Acetylcholine (ACh). ACh is released into the synaptic clefts from the pre- and the postsynaptic neurons of the parasympathetic nervous system.

In the sympathetic nervous system, what neurotransmitter is released from the preganglionic neuron into the synaptic cleft?

ACh. Remember that while the postganglionic neurotransmitters may differ between the sympathetic and parasympathetic branches of the autonomic nervous system, the preganglionic neurotransmitter released into the synaptic cleft is identical—ACh.

Where are sympathetic preganglionic fibers located?

In the paravertebral chains on either side of the spinal column or the prevertebral ganglia on the ventral surface of the aorta. Sympathetic preganglionic fibers are short.

Where are parasympathetic preganglionic fibers located?

In or near the wall of the organ they innervate. Parasympathetic preganglionic fibers are very long.

Where are nicotinic receptors located?

Postsynaptic neurons in ganglia of both the parasympathetic nervous system (PNS) and sympathetic nervous system (SNS); adrenal medulla; neuromuscular junction (NMJ); central nervous system (CNS)

Where are muscarinic receptors located?	Organs innervated by the PNS; thermoregulatory sweat glands innervated by the SNS; CNS (cortex, hippocampus)
What does the PNS do to heart rate?	It decreases the heart rate. Remember that at rest the heart is constantly under parasympathetic tone to slow the heart rate from the intrinsic rate set by the sinoatrial (SA) node at about 80 beats per minute.
What enzyme catalyzes the reaction between choline and acetyl-CoA to form ACh?	Choline acetyltransferase (CAT)
The neuronal release of ACh into the synapse is inhibited by what toxin?	*Botulinum* toxin
What organism produces *botulinum* toxin?	*Clostridium botulinum* (anaerobic, spore forming, gram-positive rod)
The venom of which spiders result in the release of stored ACh into the synapse?	Any spider of the genus *Latrodectus* (widow spiders) of which the black widow is the most common species found in North America. They produce α-latrotoxin which causes the release of ACh from the preganglionic neuron into the synaptic cleft.
What enzyme degrades ACh?	Acetylcholinesterase (AChE)
What are the breakdown products of ACh?	Choline and acetate
Where is AChE located in the autonomic nervous system?	In the synaptic cleft
What is muscarine?	It is an alkaloid found in various poisonous mushrooms.

Where are each of the following types of muscarinic receptors found in the body?

M_1	Nerves; gastric parietal cells
M_2	Nerves; cardiac cells; smooth muscle
M_3	Smooth muscle; exocrine glands; lungs; gastrointestinal (GI) tract; eye; bladder
M_4	CNS
M_5	CNS

For each of the following muscarinic receptor types, name the type of G-protein it is coupled to and the second messenger system responsible for execution of its activity upon stimulation:

M_1 — G_q coupled; inositol triphosphate (IP_3), diacylglycerol (DAG) cascade

M_2 — G_i coupled; inhibition of cyclic AMP (cAMP) production, activation of potassium channels

M_3 — G_q coupled; IP_3, DAG cascade

M_4 — G_i coupled; inhibition of cAMP production

M_5 — G_q coupled; IP_3, DAG cascade

Does the PNS directly innervate the vasculature?

No. Vascular tone is primarily determined by the degree of stimulation of adrenergic receptors of the sympathetic nervous system which directly innervate the vascular smooth muscle cells. However, there are muscarinic receptors located on the vasculature.

How can ACh lower blood pressure?

ACh binds to ACh receptors in the vasculature leading to increased synthesis of nitric oxide (NO) via second messenger pathways. An increase in NO leads to vasodilation.

NO is also known as what?

Endothelial-derived relaxation factor (EDRF)

What amino acid is a precursor to NO synthesis?

Arginine

Does AChE have a high affinity for ACh?

Yes

Does ACh increase or decrease the following (in other words, what is the effect of parasympathetic stimulation of the following)?

Blood pressure	Decreases (both arterial and venous dilation via NO)
Heart rate	Decreases (via M_2 receptors)
Salivation	Increases (via M_3 receptors)
Lacrimation	Increases (via M_3 receptors)
Sweating	Increases (via sympathetic stimulation of muscarinic cholinergic receptors)
GI secretions	Increases (via M_3 receptors)
GI motility	Increases (via M_3 receptors)
Miosis (constriction of pupil)	Increases (via M_3 receptors)
Bladder detrusor muscle tone	Increases (via M_3 receptors)
Bladder sphincter tone	Decreases (in combination with increased detrusor tone this leads to increased urination also via M_3 receptors)
Bronchodilation	Decreases (via M_3 receptors)

What does ACh do to the ciliary muscle of the eye?

Increased contraction which leads to increased accommodation

How does ACh cause miosis?

Increased contraction of the circular muscle in the iris

Does bethanechol have muscarinic activity?

Yes (agonist)

Does bethanechol have nicotinic activity?

No

Does AChE have a high affinity for bethanechol?

No (zero affinity). This gives bethanechol a long duration of action.

What is a clinical use for bethanechol?

Nonobstructive urinary retention as can result from denervation of the urinary sphincter in conditions such as diabetes or spinal cord injury. Bethanechol can also be used for gastroesophageal reflux disease (GERD). As a cholinergic drug, it will increase detrusor tone and GI motility.

Does carbachol have muscarinic activity?	Yes, it is a muscarinic agonist.
Does carbachol have nicotinic activity?	Yes, it is also a nicotinic agonist.
Does AChE have a high affinity for carbachol?	No, the enzyme has zero affinity for carbachol.
What is carbachol used for?	It is a miotic agent to reduce intraocular pressure (IOP) in emergency settings of narrow-angle and open-angle glaucoma.
Does pilocarpine have muscarinic activity?	Yes, it is a muscarinic agonist.
Does pilocarpine have nicotinic activity?	No
Does AChE have a high affinity for pilocarpine?	No, the enzyme has zero affinity for pilocarpine.
What is pilocarpine used for?	It is the miotic drug of choice to lower IOP in emergency settings of narrow-angle and open-angle glaucoma.
Can pilocarpine cross the blood-brain barrier (BBB)?	Yes. Because it is a tertiary, uncharged amine.
Give examples of reversible AChE inhibitors:	Neostigmine; pyridostigmine; physostigmine; edrophonium; rivastigmine; donepezil; galantamine; tacrine
What are donepezil, galantamine, rivastigmine, and tacrine used for?	Alzheimer-type dementia. They are AChE inhibitors, thereby increasing the levels of ACh in the brain.
What two AChE inhibitors are quaternary ammonium compounds and therefore cannot cross the BBB?	1. Neostigmine 2. Pyridostigmine As a result, these drugs will not reverse the central nervous system effects of cholinergic toxicity.
What short-acting AChE inhibitor is used to diagnose myasthenia gravis and is also used to differentiate myasthenic from cholinergic crisis?	Edrophonium. The trade name of edrophonium is Tensilon. This test is commonly referred to as the Tensilon test.

Which reversible AChE inhibitor is used as an antidote in atropine overdose?

Physostigmine, a tertiary amine, is able to cross the BBB to act on the CNS.

Give examples of irreversible AChE inhibitors:

Echothiophate; isoflurophate; sarin; malathion; parathion

Name an irreversible AChE inhibitor that is used as nerve gas:

Sarin

Which two AChE inhibitors are used as insecticides?

1. Malathion
2. Parathion

What is another name for the irreversible AChE inhibitors?

Organophosphates

How do organophosphates irreversibly inhibit AChE?

The phosphate group covalently binds to serine hydroxyl group in the active site of AChE, thereby rendering the enzyme permanently inactive.

What is used to counteract the muscarinic and CNS effects of organophosphate poisoning?

Atropine via competitive inhibition. Atropine binds the muscarinic receptors, outcompeting the increased levels of ACh thereby preventing overstimulation.

What agent is used to reactivate inhibited AChE during organophosphate poisoning?

Pralidoxime (2-PAM). It is critical to initiate treatment with pralidoxime early along with atropine to prevent the process of aging where AChE is irreversibly inactivated by the organophosphates.

What are the signs and symptoms of organophosphate poisoning?

SLUDGE: salivation; lacrimation; urination; diaphoresis; GI motility (diarrhea); emesis. Basically, parasympathetic overstimulation.

Does atropine block nicotinic receptors, muscarinic receptors, or both?

It blocks muscarinic receptors.

What are the pharmacologic actions of atropine?

Mydriasis; cycloplegia; tachycardia; sedation; urinary retention; constipation; dry mouth; dry eyes; decreased sweating; hallucinations; sedation; hyperthermia; delirium; blurred vision; coma (high doses). Basically, anticholinergic/sympathetic overstimulation.

What class of drugs can be used to counteract atropine overdose?	AChE inhibitors
Name three drug classes that may cause antimuscarinic adverse effects:	1. Sedating/first-generation antihistamines (diphenhydramine) 2. Tricyclic antidepressants (TCAs) 3. Phenothiazines
Low-dose (<0.5-1 mg) atropine does what to heart rate?	Decreases heart rate (unknown paradoxical vagalmimetic effect)
High-dose (>0.5-1 mg) atropine does what to heart rate?	Increases heart rate (parasympatholytic effect)
What is belladonna?	A perennial plant also known as "deadly nightshade" due to the toxic effects of its foliage and berries from which atropine is derived. Other toxins include scopolamine and hyoscyamine. The name belladonna derives from the cosmetic enhancing effects of dilated pupils, blushing of the cheeks, and reddening of the lips for which the plant was originally used.
How does scopolamine differ from atropine?	Scopolamine has a longer duration of action, more potent CNS effects, and is able to block short-term memory.
What is the main therapeutic indication of scopolamine?	Motion sickness
Giving drugs with anticholinergic activity can precipitate an emergent situation in patients with what medical condition?	Patients with narrow-angle glaucoma
What are the signs and symptoms of acute-angle-closure glaucoma?	General distress; pain; headache; red eye; photophobia; increased IOP; visual changes; malaise; nausea; vomiting
What two anticholinergic agents are quaternary ammonium compounds and used for the treatment of asthma and chronic obstructive pulmonary disease (COPD)?	1. Ipratropium 2. Tiotropium Tiotropium has a longer half-life compared to ipratropium.
Does ipratropium effect airway secretions?	No (unlike atropine, which decreases airway secretions)

Name three ganglionic blocking agents:	1. Hexamethonium 2. Mecamylamine 3. Trimethaphan
What are ganglionic blocking agents primarily used for?	Lowering blood pressure; blocking autonomic nervous system reflexes; smoking cessation due to blockade of central nicotine receptors
Why can ganglionic blockers cause a marked postural hypotension?	Since sympathetic tone to the blood vessels is blocked, both arterial and venous dilation occur, lowering blood pressure. Moreover, the ganglionic blockers prevent the sympathetically mediated baroreceptor response to a sudden decrease in blood pressure, such as that occurs with a rapid change in position from sitting to standing.
Neuromuscular blocking agents (NMBs) can be grouped into what two general categories?	1. Depolarizing 2. Nondepolarizing
Do NMBs work at muscarinic or nicotinic receptors?	Nicotinic receptors (remember the NMJ has nicotinic receptors).
How many subunits is the nicotinic receptor made of?	Five subunits. Two α- and three β-subunits make up this transmembrane ligand-gated ion channel.
Which subunit of the nicotinic receptor does ACh bind to?	Between the two α-subunits
Binding of ACh to the nicotinic receptor at the NMJ is required to open which type of ion channel?	Sodium channel
What is the most commonly used NMB?	Succinylcholine, the only depolarizing NMB. This is an ideal drug for endotracheal intubation due to its fast onset of action and short duration of action.
How does succinylcholine work at the NMJ?	It behaves as a cholinergic agonist that remains bound to the ACh receptor for a prolonged period.

What happens during each of the following phases of succinylcholine activity at the NMJ?

Phase I

The receptor becomes depolarized and transient fasciculations are observed as various motor units depolarize.

Phase II

The receptor becomes resistant to depolarization and a flaccid paralysis ensues.

What are the two main uses of succinylcholine?

1. It is used for facilitation of endotracheal intubation via relaxation of pharyngeal and laryngeal muscles.
2. It is used as an adjunct during electroconvulsive shock therapy to prevent prolonged full body convulsions which would result in muscle breakdown. A tourniquet is placed on a lower extremity to prevent the drug from reaching this location so that the seizure is visible in a localized area and the rest of the body is spared.

Is succinylcholine short or long acting?

It is short acting with a duration of 4-8 minutes because of rapid hydrolysis by plasma cholinesterase.

What are the adverse effects of succinylcholine?

Malignant hyperthermia; apnea; hypertension; hyperkalemia

What are the signs and symptoms of malignant hyperthermia?

Muscular rigidity; increased oxygen consumption; increased carbon dioxide production (usually the first sign detected during surgery); tachycardia; hyperthermia is a late finding

How is malignant hyperthermia treated?

With dantrolene

What is the mechanism of action of dantrolene?

It inhibits calcium release from the sarcoplasmic reticulum of muscle cells, thereby relaxing muscle tone and reducing heat production.

Succinylcholine may have a prolonged half-life in what type of patients?

Patients with a genetic deficiency or altered form of plasma cholinesterase

What is the mechanism of action of nondepolarizing NMBs?	Competitive antagonists of ACh at the NMJ
Which drug is the prototype of the nondepolarizing NMBs?	Tubocurarine
What antidote is used in tubocurarine overdose?	AChE inhibitor (increases ACh concentration which competes with tubocurarine at ACh receptors at the NMJ)
List in order, from first to last, the muscles that are paralyzed by nondepolarizing NMBs:	1. Small muscles of the face and eye 2. Fingers 3. Limbs, neck, trunk 4. Intercostals 5. Diaphragm
Which antimicrobial class of drugs may act in synergy with nondepolarizing NMBs by inhibiting release of ACh from nerve endings by competing with calcium ions, thereby increasing neuromuscular blockade?	Aminoglycosides (most likely to occur with high doses; patients with hypocalcemia, hypomagnesemia, or neuromuscular disorders)
Give examples of nondepolarizing NMBs:	Tubocurarine; atracurium; mivacurium; rocuronium; vecuronium; pancuronium; pipercuronium
What is the only nondepolarizing NMB that does not require dosage reduction in patients with renal failure?	Atracurium, which excreted in bile, not in urine
What nondepolarizing NMB has the most rapid onset of action?	Rocuronium. Think: ROcuronium— Rapid Onset
In what situations are nondepolarizing NMBs used?	Adjunct to general anesthesia to facilitate endotracheal intubation and to relax skeletal muscles during surgery; to facilitate mechanical ventilation in ICU patients

ADRENERGIC AGENTS

What are the major neurotransmitters of the SNS?	Epinephrine; norepinephrine; dopamine
What amino acid is the precursor to dopamine, epinephrine, and norepinephrine?	Tyrosine

What are the steps, in order, to the synthesis of epinephrine starting from tyrosine?

Tyrosine is converted into DOPA by tyrosine hydroxylase (rate-limiting step); DOPA is converted into dopamine by DOPA decarboxylase; dopamine is converted into norepinephrine by dopamine β-hydroxylase; norepinephrine is converted into epinephrine by methylation in the adrenal medulla.

What two enzymes metabolize norepinephrine?

1. Monoamine oxidase (MAO)
2. Catechol-*O*-methyltransferase (COMT)

What is the mechanism of action of reserpine?

It inhibits the transport of norepinephrine from the neuronal cytoplasm into the synaptic vesicles.

What are the common side effects of reserpine?

Depression; sedation

What breakdown products of norepinephrine are excreted in the urine and can be measured to help diagnose pheochromocytoma?

Vanillylmandelic acid (VMA); metanephrine; normetanephrine

What are the two major classes of adrenergic receptors?

1. α-Receptors
2. β-Receptors

What neurotransmitters are metabolized by MAO type A?

Norepinephrine; epinephrine; serotonin; tyramine; dopamine

What neurotransmitters does MAO type B metabolize?

Dopamine. Dopamine is metabolized by both the A and B type of the enzyme.

How does cocaine increase norepinephrine levels in the synaptic cleft?

It inhibits the reuptake of neurotransmitter back into the presynaptic neuron.

How do amphetamine, ephedrine, and tyramine increase norepinephrine levels?

They act as indirect sympathomimetic agents by entering the presynaptic neuron releasing stored norepinephrine into the synaptic cleft.

Where are α₁-receptors found?

Vascular smooth muscle; papillary dilator muscle; pilomotor smooth muscle; prostate; heart

Where are α₂-receptors found?

Postsynaptic CNS adrenoceptors; pancreatic β-cells; platelets; adrenergic and cholinergic nerve terminals; vascular smooth muscle; fat cells

Where are β_1-receptors found?	Heart; juxtaglomerular cells
Where are β_2-receptors found?	Respiratory, uterine, and vascular smooth muscle; skeletal muscle; liver
Where are D_1-receptors found?	Smooth muscle
Where are D_2-receptors found?	Nerve endings
Compare and contrast the local versus the systemic effects of α_2-receptor activation.	Local infusion of an α_2-agonist will activate the α_2-receptors in the vasculature, causing vasoconstriction. Systemic administration will activate the central α_2-receptors in the locus ceruleus which inhibits norepinephrine release and sympathetic activation. The central effects overwhelm the local effects leading to decreased blood pressure.
Give examples of α_2-receptor agonists:	Clonidine; α-methyldopa; guanabenz; guanfacine; dexmedetomidine
What are the therapeutic indications of clonidine?	Hypertension; severe pain; heroin withdrawal; nicotine withdrawal; ethanol dependence; clozapine-induced sialorrhea; prevention of migraines
What is dexmedetomidine used for?	Sedation of intubated and mechanically ventilated patients; prolongation of spinal anesthesia
With drugs that activate both α- and β-receptors, which receptors are generally activated first (which receptors are more sensitive)?	β-Receptors
Activation of what receptor type in the eye will lead to contraction of the radial muscle and subsequently lead to mydriasis?	α_1-Receptor
For each of the following receptor types, name the type of G-protein it is coupled to:	
α_1	G_q
α_2	G_i
β_1, β_2, D_1	G_s

Name the major effects mediated by each of the following receptor types:

α_1

Mydriasis; vasoconstriction → increased blood pressure; decreased urination; increased glycogenolysis; decreased renin release; ejaculation

α_2

Inhibition of norepinephrine release (central effect); inhibition of insulin release; platelet aggregation

β_1

Increased heart rate; increased conduction velocity; increased force of heart contraction; increased renin release

β_2

Vasodilation; bronchodilation; relaxation of uterine, respiratory, and vascular smooth muscle; increased insulin secretion; increased potassium uptake; increased glycogenolysis

Peripheral D_1

Vasodilation of coronary, renal, and mesenteric vasculature; increased glomerular filtration rate (GFR); increased renal blood flow (RBF); increased sodium excretion

Will α_2-receptor activation in the pancreas cause insulin secretion to increase or decrease?

It will cause insulin secretion to decrease.

Will β_2-receptor activation in the pancreas cause insulin secretion to increase or decrease?

It will cause insulin secretion to increase.

Which receptor type does epinephrine preferentially bind to at low doses?

β-Receptors (vasodilation in vasculature)

Which receptor type does epinephrine preferentially bind to at high doses?

α-Receptors (vasoconstriction in vasculature)

What is the drug of choice in patients with type 1 (immediate) hypersensitivity reactions?

Epinephrine

What is the dose of epinephrine given for anaphylaxis?

0.1-0.5 mg. Note: The EpiPen (epinephrine auto-injector) that many patients with a history of anaphylaxis carry is 0.3 mg.

What is the concentration of epinephrine used for anaphylaxis?

1:1000

What is the concentration of epinephrine used for advanced cardiac life support (ACLS) protocol?	1:10,000
Why is epinephrine often given in combination with local anesthetics?	Epinephrine causes a vasoconstriction, thereby inhibiting the local anesthetics redistribution away from its site of action, so it increases the duration of local anesthesia.
What is the concentration of epinephrine when given in combination with local anesthetics?	1:100,000

State whether each of the following cardiovascular effects increases or decreases with low-dose epinephrine:

Peripheral vascular resistance	Decreases
Systolic blood pressure	Increases
Diastolic blood pressure	Decreases
Pulse pressure	Increases
What receptors are activated by isoproterenol?	$\beta_1 = \beta_2$
What receptors are activated by dopamine?	$D > \beta > \alpha$
What receptors are activated by dobutamine?	$\beta_1 > \beta_2$
What receptors are activated by phenylephrine?	$\alpha_1 > \alpha_2$
Does norepinephrine activate β_2-receptors?	No
Activation of dopamine receptors will cause what type of response in the mesenteric and renal vasculature?	Vasodilation
What is dopamine metabolized to?	Homovanillic acid (HVA)
What is dobutamine used for?	Increases cardiac output in congestive heart failure (CHF) without affecting RBF (unlike dopamine)
Tyramine is a breakdown product of which amino acid?	Tyrosine

Where is tyramine found?	Examples of foods and beverages which contain tyramine include: beer, ale, robust red wines, chianti, vermouth, homemade breads, cheese, sour cream, bananas, red plums, figs, raisins, avocados, fava beans, Italian broad beans, green bean pods, eggplant, pickled herring, liver, dry sausages, canned meats, salami, yogurt, soup cubes, commercial gravies, chocolate, and soy sauce.
What enzyme is responsible for the breakdown of tyramine?	MAO type A
What can potentially happen if a patient on a monoamine oxidase inhibitor (MAOI) consumes large amount of fermented cheese?	Hypertensive crisis due to tyramine in the cheese which leads to the release of norepinephrine from storage vesicles in presynaptic neurons
What is phenylephrine and pseudoephedrine used to treat?	Nasal congestion
What are mixed action adrenergic agonists?	Substances that release stored norepinephrine from nerve terminals and also directly stimulate α and β-receptors
What are some examples of mixed action adrenergic agonists?	Ephedrine; pseudoephedrine; metaraminol
Which drug is a nonselective, competitive antagonist at both α_1- and α_2-receptors?	Phentolamine
Which drug is a nonselective, irreversible antagonist at both α_1- and α_2-receptors?	Phenoxybenzamine
What are phentolamine and phenoxybenzamine mainly used for?	To achieve α-receptor blockade before surgical removal of pheochromocytoma, to achieve perioperative blood pressure control, and to prevent intraoperative hypertension from release of catecholamines during surgical manipulation
What is the mechanism of action of prazosin?	Selective α_1-antagonist
What are prazosin, terazosin, and doxazosin used to treat?	Benign prostatic hyperplasia (BPH); hypertension

Does the "H" in BPH stand for hypertrophy or hyperplasia?

Hyperplasia, though hypertrophy is still sometimes erroneously used. There is an actual increase in the number of prostatic cells in BPH. The cells do not simply increase in volume as do, for example, skeletal or cardiac muscle cells in response to increased used.

This drug is a selective α_{1A}-receptor antagonist, used in the treatment of BPH, and has less cardiovascular side effects versus traditional α_1-antagonists.

Tamsulosin

What advantages do selective α_1-antagonists have over nonselective α-antagonists?

Less reflex tachycardia

What CNS prejunctional α_2-receptor antagonist is used to treat postural hypotension and erectile dysfunction (impotence)?

Yohimbine

What CNS prejunctional α_2-receptor antagonist is used to treat depression?

Mirtazapine

Give examples of β_1-selective antagonists:

Acebutolol; atenolol; bisoprolol; betaxolol; esmolol; metoprolol

Give examples of nonselective β-antagonists:

Propranolol; timolol; pindolol; nadolol

Give examples of mixed α_1/β-antagonists:

Carvedilol; labetalol

What is the name of a β-antagonist that also blocks potassium channels and is used as an antiarrhythmic?

Sotalol

What is intrinsic sympathomimetic activity (ISA)?

Drugs act as partial agonists and only work when there is increased sympathetic drive such as with exercise; less bradycardia; less effects on lipid metabolism

Which two β-antagonists have ISA?

1. Acebutolol
2. Pindolol

What happens to exercise tolerance in patients being treated with β-blockers?

Decreased exercise tolerance

What are the main therapeutic indications of β-blockers?	Angina; arrhythmias; hypertension; CHF (not all β-blockers); thyrotoxicosis; glaucoma (ophthalmic formulations)
What are some noncardiovascular uses of propranolol?	Migraine prophylaxis; performance anxiety "stage fright"
β-Blockers can inhibit the majority of effects caused by thyrotoxicosis except for what sign?	Diaphoresis. Remember that sweat glands have muscarinic receptors and are cholinergic rather than adrenergic.
β-Blockers can inhibit the majority of effects caused by hypoglycemia except for what sign?	Diaphoresis. β-Blockers are contraindicated in diabetic patients treated with oral hypoglycemics for this reason.
What does propranolol do to serum triglycerides?	Increases serum triglycerides
What does propranolol do to serum low-density lipoprotein (LDL)?	Increases serum LDL
Why does propranolol cause vivid dreams?	Crosses the BBB
Why should β-blockers be tapered down instead of abruptly discontinued?	Chronic therapy leads to upregulation of β-receptors; therefore, abrupt discontinuation may lead to life-threatening cardiovascular rebound effects (tachycardia; hypertension; arrhythmias; death)

CLINICAL VIGNETTES

A mother brings her 4-month-old infant to the pediatrician. The child developed what appeared to be a viral febrile illness which rapidly progressed. The infant now appears listless and has decreased muscle tone. The mother reports decreased feeding and bowel movements and says that the child's cry sounds different from normal. The only treatment she has initiated is warm milk with honey to help the child's immune system. What is the most likely diagnosis?

While the child may have initially had a viral upper respiratory tract infection (URI), ingestion of honey exposed the infant to *C. botulinum* spores which are able to colonize the immature pediatric small intestines. Botulinum toxin is then released into the systemic circulation which blocks the release of ACh from the synaptic cleft, leading to the flaccid paralysis known as "floppy baby syndrome."

A patient has been found to inconsistently have elevated blood pressure during various office visits over the past several years. A decision is made to try propranolol to control the patient's blood pressure. On return visit 2 weeks later, the patient's blood pressure is markedly elevated and the patient reports headaches and blurred vision. What is the most likely diagnosis?

Pheochromocytoma. The patient most likely had sporadic release of catecholamines from the tumor leading to periods of increased blood pressure. The most common neurotransmitter released from pheochromocytomas is norepinephrine. Nonselective blockade of the β-adrenergic receptors by propranolol leads to unopposed α-adrenergic receptor activation by the norepinephrine released by the pheochromocytoma leading to a hypertensive emergency.

A 62-year-old man comes to his primary care physician for a regular checkup. His blood pressure has been mildly elevated on the last two office visits. Today's reading is 140/92. He is also complaining of some difficulty initiating urination as well as getting up two or more times per night to urinate. What is the best pharmacotherapy to initiate at this time?

Prazosin or another selective α_1-antagonist such as terazosin or doxazosin. Prazosin blocks α_1-receptors found in the base of the bladder and prostate, preventing constriction and decreasing the resistance to urine flow. It also relaxes vascular smooth muscle leading to decreased blood pressure. Always try to minimize the amount of medications you prescribe for patients. Here, the dual action of prazosin makes it an ideal choice for this patient with two separate health concerns.

CHAPTER 5

CNS Agents

GENERAL AND LOCAL ANESTHETICS

State which stage of anesthesia each of the following descriptions refers to?

Delirium; violent behavior; increased blood pressure; increased respiratory rate; irregular breathing rate and volume; amnesia; retching and vomiting with stimulation; disconjugate gaze

Stage II (excitement)

Depression of vasomotor center; depression of respiratory center; death may occur

Stage IV (medullary depression)

Eye movements cease; fixed pupils; regular respiration; relaxation of skeletal muscles

Stage III (surgical anesthesia)

Loss of pain sensation; patient is conscious; no amnesia in early part of this stage

Stage I (analgesia)

Give examples of inhaled anesthetics:

Halothane; nitrous oxide; isoflurane; enflurane; sevoflurane; desflurane; methoxyflurane

With regard to inhaled anesthetics, what does MAC stand for?

Minimum alveolar concentration. Note: this is not to be confused with monitored anesthesia care also commonly referred to as MAC, which is a combination of regional anesthesia, sedation, and analgesia.

What is MAC in regard to inhaled anesthetics?

The concentration of inhaled anesthetic required to stop movement in 50% of patients given a standardized skin incision; a measure of potency for inhaled anesthetics

For potent inhaled anesthetics, is the MAC small or large?

Small (inverse of the MAC is used as an index of potency for inhaled anesthetics)

Which inhaled anesthetic has the largest MAC?

Nitrous oxide (>100%)

Which inhaled anesthetic has the smallest MAC?

Halothane (0.75%)

As lipid solubility of an inhaled anesthetic increases, what happens to the concentration of inhaled anesthetic needed to produce anesthesia, that is, does it increase or decrease?

It decreases.

What is the blood/gas partition coefficient?

The ratio of the total amount of gas in the blood relative to the gas equilibrium phase. It refers to an inhaled anesthetic's solubility in the blood.

If an inhaled anesthetic has a high blood/gas partition coefficient, will times of induction and recovery be increased or decreased?

It will be increased because the time to increase arterial tension is longer.

Give an example of an inhaled anesthetic with a low blood/gas partition coefficient (low blood solubility):

Nitrous oxide (0.5); desflurane (0.4)

Give an example of an inhaled anesthetic with a high blood/gas partition coefficient (high blood solubility):

Halothane (2.3); enflurane (1.8)

Which inhaled anesthetic, halothane or nitrous oxide, will take longer to change the depth of anesthesia when the concentration of the inhaled anesthetic has been changed?

Halothane

Are MAC values additive?

Yes

Are MAC values higher or lower in elderly patients?

They are lower, thus elderly patients generally require lower concentrations of inhaled anesthetics.

Are MAC values higher or lower when opioid analgesics and/or sedative hypnotics are used concomitantly?

They are lower.

Do inhaled anesthetics increase or decrease the response to P_{CO_2} levels?	Decrease
Do inhaled anesthetics increase or decrease cerebral vascular flow?	Increase
Do inhaled anesthetics increase or decrease intracranial pressure?	Increase
Do inhaled anesthetics relax or strengthen uterine smooth muscle contractions?	Relax (except methoxyflurane when briefly inhaled, therefore, can be used during childbirth)
Which of the inhaled anesthetics is not a halogenated hydrocarbon?	Nitrous oxide
Are the inhaled halogenated hydrocarbon anesthetics volatile or nonvolatile gases?	Volatile gases
Which inhaled anesthetic is associated with malignant hyperthermia?	Halothane
What characterizes malignant hyperthermia?	Hyperthermia; muscle rigidity; acidosis; hypertension; hyperkalemia
Should a patient with a family history positive for malignant hyperthermia be concerned?	Yes, because a genetic defect in ryanodine receptors may be inherited.
What drug is given to treat malignant hyperthermia?	Dantrolene
Which inhaled anesthetic is associated with increased bronchiolar secretions?	Isoflurane
Which inhaled anesthetic is associated with hepatitis?	Halothane
Halothane is not hepatotoxic in what patient population?	Pediatric patients
Which inhaled anesthetic is the least hepatotoxic?	Nitrous oxide
Which inhaled anesthetic is associated with increased bronchiolar spasms?	Isoflurane
Which inhaled anesthetic relaxes bronchial smooth muscle?	Halothane

Which inhaled anesthetic is associated with cardiac arrhythmias?	Halothane
Which inhaled anesthetics increase heart rate (via reflex secondary to vasodilation)?	Isoflurane; desflurane
Which inhaled anesthetics decrease heart rate?	Halothane; enflurane; sevoflurane
Which inhaled anesthetic decreases renal and hepatic blood flow?	Halothane
Give examples of intravenous (IV) anesthetics:	Propofol; fentanyl; ketamine; midazolam; thiopental; etomidate
Which of the previously mentioned IV anesthetics is a barbiturate?	Thiopental
Which of the previously mentioned IV anesthetics is a benzodiazepine?	Midazolam
Which of the previously mentioned IV anesthetics is an opioid?	Fentanyl
Is thiopental used for induction, maintenance, or both?	Induction
Pharmacodynamically, how does recovery occur with the rapid-acting barbiturates?	Rapid redistribution from the central nervous system (CNS) to peripheral tissues
State whether thiopental increases, decreases, or does not change each of the following physiologic effects:	
Cerebral blood flow	No change
Respiratory function	Decreases
Blood pressure	Decreases
Why should caution be taken when administering thiopental to asthmatic patients?	May cause laryngospasm
Midazolam offers which type of amnesia making it useful for monitored anesthesia care?	Anterograde amnesia
What is the antidote for midazolam-induced respiratory depression?	Flumazenil, which is also the antidote for any benzodiazepine overdose

What adverse drug reaction may be caused by fentanyl when given intravenously?	Chest wall rigidity
Does propofol have good analgesic properties?	No
About which allergies should a patient be questioned before administration of propofol?	Egg and soybeans. Propofol is prepared as a lipid emulsion using egg and soybean lecithin. This gives propofol its white color and can cause allergic reactions in patients with sensitivities to these substances.
Does propofol increase or decrease blood pressure?	It decreases blood pressure.
Is propofol used for induction, maintenance, or both?	It is used for both.
Which IV anesthetic causes dissociative anesthesia?	Ketamine
What is dissociative anesthesia?	The patient is unconscious and feels no pain, yet appears awake. Eyes may open and the swallowing reflex is present, but the patient is sedated, immobile, and usually amnestic. Hallucinations and delirium are common.
Which anesthetic has antiemetic properties?	Propofol
Which IV anesthetic is a cardiovascular stimulant (increases blood pressure and cardiac output)?	Ketamine
Which IV anesthetic causes vivid dreams and hallucinations?	Ketamine
Does ketamine increase or decrease cerebral blood flow?	Increase
What is the most cardiac-stable IV anesthetic agent?	Etomidate
Are local anesthetics weak acids or weak bases?	Weak bases

Give examples of amide local anesthetics:

Lidocaine; prilocaine; articaine; mepivacaine; bupivacaine (all have >1 "i" in their generic name)

Give examples of ester local anesthetics:

Cocaine; benzocaine; procaine (all have only one "i" in their generic name)

Which medication, when used in combination, reduces systemic toxicity and increases the duration of action of local anesthetics?

Epinephrine, by inducing a local vasoconstriction

Epinephrine should not be combined with local anesthetics when injecting near which anatomic sites?

Digits; nose; ears; penis; and any end-artery circulation

Which type of enzymes metabolize amide local anesthetics and where are they located?

Amidases located in the liver

Which type of enzymes metabolize ester local anesthetics and where are they located?

Esterases located in tissues and blood

What is the mechanism of action of local anesthetics?

Inhibition of sodium channels in axonal membranes via binding to the channels in their inactivated state and preventing a structural change to the resting state

Do local anesthetics need to be in the ionized or nonionized form to bind to the sodium channel?

Ionized form

Do local anesthetics need to be in the ionized or nonionized form to gain access to the sodium channel, which is located on the inner side of the axonal membrane?

Nonionized form (must be able to cross lipophilic axonal membrane)

All local anesthetics cause vasodilation with the exception of which drug?

Cocaine (causes vasoconstriction)

Nerve fibers most sensitive to blockade are of smaller or larger diameter?

Smaller diameter

Nerve fibers most sensitive to blockade have low or high firing rates?

High firing rates

Which nerve fibers are most sensitive to local anesthetics?

Type B fibers; type C fibers

Which nerve fibers are least sensitive to local anesthetics?	Type A α-fibers
What are the adverse effects of local anesthetics?	Hypotension (except cocaine); nystagmus; seizures; dizziness; allergic reactions (rare)
Allergic reactions are more associated with ester or amide local anesthetics?	Esters (via para-aminobenzoic acid [PABA] formation)

OPIOID ANALGESICS AND ANTAGONISTS

Which neurotransmitter binds to the δ-opioid receptor?	Enkephalin
Which neurotransmitter binds to the κ-opioid receptor?	Dynorphin
Which neurotransmitter binds to the μ-opioid receptor?	β-Endorphin
What is the mechanism of action of medications that activate *presynaptic* opioid receptors?	Inhibits calcium influx through voltage-gated ion channels, thereby inhibiting neurotransmitter release
What is the mechanism of action of medications that activate *postsynaptic* opioid receptors?	Increases potassium efflux from cells leading to membrane hyperpolarization and thereby inhibition of neurotransmitter release
Opioid receptors are coupled to what type of proteins?	Inhibitory G-proteins (inhibits adenylyl cyclase)
What is the prototype opioid analgesic?	Morphine
Why must caution be taken when using opioids in patients with head injuries?	Opioids may increase intracranial pressure
Where in the midbrain are opioid receptors located?	Periaqueductal gray region (binding to these receptors leads to activation of descending pathways to the raphe nuclei, thereby decreasing transmission throughout pain pathways)
Where in the dorsal horn of the spinal cord are opioid receptors located?	Primary afferent fibers (binding to these receptors leads to inhibition of substance P release)

Are opioid analgesics better at relieving intermittent or persistent pain?

Persistent pain

What is the mechanism of morphine-induced hypotension and pruritus?

Increased histamine release from mast cells

Do opioid analgesics increase or decrease gastrointestinal (GI) peristalsis?

Decrease (they cause constipation)

Which two opioids are used specifically to treat diarrhea?

1. Loperamide
2. Diphenoxylate

Which opioid analgesic does not increase the tone of the biliary tract, bladder, and ureter?

Meperidine (antagonizes muscarinic receptors)

Do opioid analgesics increase or decrease uterine contractions during pregnancy?

They decrease uterine contractions, thus a good contraction pattern should be achieved before placement of an epidural catheter during labor.

Do opioid analgesics cause miosis or mydriasis of the pupils?

Miosis (common sign of opioid overdose is pinpoint pupils)

What is the mechanism of opioid-induced miosis?

Increased parasympathetic (cholinergic) activity in the pupilary constrictor muscles

Which opioid analgesic does not cause miosis?

Meperidine (antagonizes muscarinic receptors)

Which two opioids are used specifically to treat cough?

1. Codeine
2. Dextromethorphan

Opioids suppress the cough reflex.

Is dextromethorphan a natural or synthetic opioid?

Synthetic

What is the mechanism of opioid-induced urinary retention?

Increases antidiuretic hormone (ADH)

Do opioid analgesics promote emesis or act as antiemetics?

Promote emesis

What is the mechanism of opioid-induced emesis?

Activation of the chemoreceptor trigger zone (CTZ)

Where is the CTZ located?

Area postrema

What is the mechanism of opioid-induced respiratory depression?	Reduced sensitivity of respiratory center to carbon dioxide levels
What is the most common cause of death in opioid overdose?	Respiratory depression
What are the two most lipophilic opioids?	1. Heroin 2. Fentanyl These two medications rapidly cross the blood-brain barrier (BBB) to produce euphoric effects.
Which opioid is the least lipophilic?	Morphine
Is morphine metabolized via phase I or phase II reactions?	Phase II metabolism (glucuronidation)
Does morphine-3-glucuronide have analgesic activity?	No
Does morphine-6-glucuronide have analgesic activity?	Yes
Which two opioid-induced effects do patients not develop tolerance to?	1. Constipation 2. Miosis
What are the signs and symptoms of opioid withdrawal?	Lacrimation; rhinorrhea; diaphoresis; yawning; goose bumps; anxiety; muscle spasms; diarrhea; increased pain sensation
Which medication is used to counteract the respiratory depression seen in opioid overdose?	IV naloxone (may need to give multiple doses as naloxone has a shorter half-life than morphine)
What is the mechanism of action of naloxone?	μ-Receptor antagonist
Which opioid antagonist is given orally to decrease cravings in alcoholism?	Naltrexone
Which opioid analgesic is used to prevent withdrawal symptoms in patients discontinuing heroin use?	Methadone
Which central-acting α_2-agonist is used to prevent withdrawal symptoms in patients discontinuing heroin use?	Clonidine

Give examples of strong opioid agonists:

Morphine; fentanyl; heroin; methadone; meperidine; hydrocodone; hydromorphone

Give examples of weak opioid agonists:

Codeine; propoxyphene

Give examples of partial opioid agonists:

Buprenorphine; pentazocine

Propoxyphene is a derivative of which opioid analgesic?

Methadone

Name two synthetic opioid analgesics:

1. Meperidine
2. Methadone

Fentanyl is chemically related to which synthetic opioid analgesic?

Meperidine

Does morphine have a high or low oral bioavailability?

Low

Which two opioids should not be given in combination with monoamine oxidase inhibitors (MAOIs)?

1. Meperidine
2. Dextromethorphan

These combinations may produce serotonin syndrome.

What drug do you get by acetylating morphine?

Heroin

Is codeine itself an active opioid analgesic?

No (must be metabolized via cytochrome P-450 2D6 to active morphine)

Which medication is commonly given in combination with codeine for the treatment of pain?

Acetaminophen

ANXIOLYTIC AND SEDATIVE-HYPNOTIC AGENTS

For each of the following sedative-hypnotic-induced CNS effects, place in order from effect caused by lowest to highest dose of drug: coma; anesthesia; hypnosis; sedation/anxiolysis; medullary depression.

Sedation/anxiolysis; hypnosis; anesthesia; medullary depression; coma

What is the first step in ethanol metabolism?

Alcohol dehydrogenase converts ethanol to acetaldehyde.

What is the second step in ethanol metabolism?	Acetaldehyde dehydrogenase converts acetaldehyde to acetate.
What enzyme does disulfiram inhibit?	Acetaldehyde dehydrogenase, leading to a build up of acetaldehyde
Which metabolite of ethanol is responsible for causing headache, hypotension, nausea, and vomiting ("hangover")?	Acetaldehyde
What does GABA stand for?	Gamma-aminobutyric acid
How many subunits make up the GABA receptor?	Five subunits
Which subunit does GABA bind to?	α-Subunit
Which subunit on the GABA receptor do benzodiazepines bind to?	γ-Subunit (binding potentiates the affinity of the GABA receptor for GABA; does not activate the receptor alone without GABA)
Which subunit on the GABA receptor do barbiturates bind to?	β-Subunit (binding potentiates the affinity of the GABA receptor for GABA; does not activate the receptor alone without GABA)
What physiologic process takes place when GABA binds to the GABA$_A$ receptor?	Increased chloride ion influx into cells leading to membrane hyperpolarization and subsequent decreased neuronal firing
What physiologic process takes place when GABA binds to the GABA$_B$ receptor?	Increased potassium ion efflux out of cells leading to membrane hyperpolarization and subsequent decreased neuronal firing
What medication binds specifically to the GABA$_B$ receptor?	Baclofen
What is baclofen used for?	Muscle relaxation
Do benzodiazepines potentiate GABA by increasing the duration or frequency of chloride ion channel opening?	Frequency
Do barbiturates potentiate GABA by increasing the duration or frequency of chloride ion channel opening?	Duration

Name three nonbenzodiazepine sleep aids that specifically bind to the BZ₁-receptor subtype:

1. Eszopiclone
2. Zolpidem
3. Zaleplon

Does zolpidem display anticonvulsant, antianxiety, or muscle relaxant properties?

No, it is a selective hypnotic along with zaleplon and eszopiclone.

Do benzodiazepines have good analgesic properties?

No

What types of actions do benzodiazepines display?

Muscle relaxant; anticonvulsant; antianxiety; sedative-hypnotic; anterograde amnesia (midazolam); alcohol withdrawal

Give examples of benzodiazepines:

Diazepam; lorazepam; alprazolam; chlordiazepoxide; clonazepam; clorazepate; midazolam; flurazepam; flunitrazepam; temazepam; triazolam; oxazepam

What is the name of the prototype benzodiazepine?

Chlordiazepoxide

What benzodiazepine is colloquially referred to as the "date rape" drug and is illegal in the United States?

Flunitrazepam (trade name: Rohypnol; slang: "roofies")

Which benzodiazepine is the longest acting?

Diazepam

Which benzodiazepine is the shortest acting?

Midazolam

What three benzodiazepines undergo phase II metabolism?

1. Lorazepam
2. Oxazepam
3. Temazepam

Which benzodiazepines are commonly used as anticonvulsants?

Diazepam; clonazepam

Which benzodiazepines are commonly used to treat alcohol withdrawal?

Oxazepam; lorazepam; diazepam; chlordiazepoxide

Which benzodiazepines are commonly used as sleep aids?

Temazepam; triazolam; flurazepam

Which benzodiazepines are commonly used as anxiolytics?

Diazepam; lorazepam; alprazolam

Why is alprazolam not the drug of choice when treating patients with chronic anxiety?	It has a short half-life, and therefore may cause withdrawal symptoms, such as anxiety, which subsequently worsens the condition and leads to higher addiction rates.
Give examples of long-acting benzodiazepines (duration of action of 1-3 d):	Diazepam; chlordiazepoxide; flurazepam; clorazepate
Give examples of intermediate-acting benzodiazepines (duration of action of 10-20 h):	Lorazepam; temazepam; alprazolam
Give examples of short-acting benzodiazepines (duration of action of 3-8 h):	Midazolam; oxazepam; triazolam
Give examples of benzodiazepine withdrawal signs and symptoms:	Insomnia; anxiety; agitation; seizures; restlessness; confusion
What are the adverse effects of benzodiazepines?	Confusion; drowsiness; ataxia; cognitive impairment; amnesia; respiratory depression
Is withdrawal more likely to occur with long-acting or short-acting benzodiazepines?	Short-acting benzodiazepines (abrupt withdrawal may ensue as drug levels are rapidly decreased versus long-acting benzodiazepines which offer a "self-tapering" mechanism which decreases the chance of withdrawal)
What is the antidote for benzodiazepine-induced CNS depression?	Flumazenil (short half-life; therefore, multiple administrations may be necessary)
What is the mechanism of action of flumazenil?	Benzodiazepine receptor antagonist
Will flumazenil decrease the effects of barbiturates?	No (barbiturates act at a different GABA receptor subtype than benzodiazepines)
Which two sedative-hypnotic drug classes are potentially fatal with overdose and/or withdrawal?	1. Barbiturates 2. Alcohols Benzodiazepines may be potentially fatal but to a lesser extent than barbiturates and alcohols.
Give examples of long-acting barbiturates (duration of action of 1-2 d):	Phenobarbital; pentobarbital

Give examples of short-acting barbiturates (duration of action of 3-8 h):	Amobarbital; secobarbital
Give an example of an ultra-short-acting barbiturate (duration of action of 30 min):	Thiopental
What is phenobarbital commonly used to treat?	Seizures (generalized tonic-clonic and partial seizures)
What is thiopental commonly used for?	Induction of anesthesia
What are short-acting barbiturates commonly used for?	Sedation; hypnosis
What kind of drug interactions can barbiturates produce?	Induction of cytochrome P-450 enzymes
What are the adverse effects of barbiturates?	Drowsiness; impair cognitive function (especially in pediatric patients); "hangover" effect; nausea; dizziness; increase heme synthesis (contraindicated in patients with acute intermittent porphyria); coma; respiratory depression; cardiovascular depression; addiction
Give examples of barbiturate withdrawal signs and symptoms:	Insomnia; tremors; anxiety; restlessness; nausea; vomiting; seizures; cardiac arrest; delirium; hyperreflexia; agitation
What drug class is used to prevent barbiturate withdrawal?	Long-acting benzodiazepines
Over-the-counter (OTC) sleep aids have what types of medications in them?	Sedating antihistamines
Give examples of sedating antihistamines:	Diphenhydramine; doxylamine; hydroxyzine (prescription only)
Give examples of antidepressants that have been used for sedation and hypnosis:	Trazodone; amitriptyline
Which medication is a partial agonist at 5-HT$_{1A}$ receptors and is effective in treating generalized anxiety disorder?	Buspirone

Does buspirone have anticonvulsant and muscle relaxant properties?	No
Is buspirone sedating?	No
How long does it take for buspirone to exert its anxiolytic effects?	1 to 2 weeks (therefore, not useful in treating an acute anxiety attack)
What types of withdrawal signs and symptoms does buspirone cause?	None

ANTIDEPRESSANT AGENTS

According to the biogenic amine theory, depression is due to a deficiency of which two neurotransmitters in the brain?	1. Serotonin (5-HT) 2. Norepinephrine (NE)
MAO_A inactivates which neurotransmitters?	5-HT; NE
MAO_B inactivates which neurotransmitter?	Dopamine (DA)
What is the mechanism of action of MAOIs?	Inactivation of MAO, thereby increasing levels of 5-HT, NE, and DA in presynaptic neurons with subsequent leakage of neurotransmitter into the synaptic cleft
Name three nonselective MAOIs:	1. Tranylcypromine 2. Phenelzine 3. Isocarboxazid
Selegiline is commonly used in the treatment of which disease?	Parkinson disease
MAO_A also inactivates which monoamine commonly found in certain cheeses (aged), alcoholic beverages, fish, chocolates, red wines, and processed meats?	Tyramine (inactivated by MAO in the GI tract)
MAOIs are the drugs of choice for treating what type of depression?	Atypical depression
How long does it take to see antidepressant effects in patients who are started on an MAOI?	2 to 4 weeks

How long should a patient wait from the time of discontinuing an MAOI to the time of starting a new antidepressant medication?	At least 2 weeks
What are the adverse effects of MAOIs?	Orthostatic hypotension; xerostomia; blurred vision; drowsiness; constipation; urinary retention
What life-threatening condition may develop when MAOIs and selective serotonin reuptake inhibitors (SSRIs) are used concomitantly?	Serotonin syndrome
What characterizes serotonin syndrome?	Rigidity; diaphoresis; hyperthermia; seizures; autonomic instability; myoclonus
What life-threatening condition may develop when patients taking MAOIs ingest foods containing tyramine?	Hypertensive crisis
What characterizes hypertensive crisis?	Hypertension; headache; tachycardia; nausea; vomiting; stroke; cardiac arrhythmias
A serotonin-like syndrome may develop when MAOIs are used concomitantly with what common OTC medication used to suppress cough?	Dextromethorphan
A serotonin-like syndrome may develop when MAOIs are used concomitantly with which opioid analgesic?	Meperidine
What is the mechanism of action of tricyclic antidepressants (TCAs)?	Inhibits reuptake of 5-HT and NE into presynaptic neurons, thereby increasing neurotransmitter concentrations in the synaptic cleft
What other types of neurotransmitter and hormonal receptors, other than 5-HT and NE, are inhibited by TCAs?	Muscarinic; α-adrenergic; histaminergic
How long does it take to see antidepressant effects in patients who are started on a TCA?	4 to 6 weeks

Give examples of TCAs:	Amitriptyline; imipramine; clomipramine; nortriptyline; protriptyline; desipramine; doxepin
What is the name of the active metabolite of amitriptyline that selectively inhibits NE reuptake?	Nortriptyline
What is the name of the active metabolite of imipramine that selectively inhibits NE reuptake?	Desipramine
Which TCA is also used for the treatment of certain types of neuropathic pain and for the prevention of migraine headaches?	Amitriptyline
Which TCA is commonly used to treat obsessive-compulsive disorder (OCD)?	Clomipramine
Which TCA is also used to treat pediatric nocturnal enuresis?	Imipramine
Why is imipramine used for childhood enuresis?	Increases contraction of internal sphincter of bladder; decreases stage 3 and 4 sleep
What are the adverse effects of the TCAs?	Xerostomia; blurred vision; urinary retention; constipation; precipitation of acute glaucoma attacks; cardiac arrhythmias; seizures (lowers seizure threshold); orthostatic hypotension with reflex tachycardia; sedation; serotonin syndrome when combined with MAOIs and/or SSRIs; coma
What are the "3 C's" of TCA toxicity?	Coma, convulsions, and cardiotoxicity
Compare TCA toxicity to SSRI toxicity.	SSRI toxicity is much lower than that seen with TCAs, and mortality is most often reported only when SSRIs are used in combination with another agent, such as alcohol. This is in contrast to TCAs, which can lead to death at much lower concentrations as compared to SSRIs.
What is the treatment for TCA overdose?	Activated charcoal to absorb the drug in the GI tract; sodium bicarbonate to correct acidosis and cardiac arrhythmias; phenytoin; magnesium

What is the mechanism of action of trazodone and nefazodone?	Inhibits reuptake of 5-HT into presynaptic neurons, thereby increasing neurotransmitter concentrations in the synaptic cleft
What adverse effect is unique to trazodone?	Priapism
What is the mechanism of action of bupropion?	Weak inhibitor of DA, 5-HT, and NE reuptake
Bupropion is also used in what settings (other than depression)?	Smoking cessation; OCD
Does bupropion cause sexual dysfunction?	No, making it a useful alternative in patients that experience sexual dysfunction with other antidepressant medications such as SSRIs
Is bupropion safe to use in patients with epilepsy?	No, because it lowers the seizure threshold.
What is the mechanism of action of mirtazapine?	α_2-Adrenoceptor antagonist (results in increased release of NE and 5-HT)
What is the major side effect of mirtazapine?	Weight gain via appetite stimulation (may be beneficial in depressed patients who become anorexic)
Name an α_2-antagonist that is used in the treatment of erectile dysfunction:	Yohimbine
What is the mechanism of action of venlafaxine?	Potent inhibitor of 5-HT and NE reuptake; weak inhibitor of DA reuptake
What is the major side effect of venlafaxine?	Hypertension
What is the mechanism of action of duloxetine?	Selective serotonin and norepinephrine reuptake inhibitor (SSNRI)
Give examples of SSRIs:	Fluoxetine; paroxetine; fluvoxamine; sertraline; citalopram; escitalopram
What is the prototype of the SSRI drug class?	Fluoxetine
What is the longest-acting SSRI?	Fluoxetine

Fluoxetine is also used in what settings (other than depression)?	Premenstrual dysphoric disorder (PMDD); bulimia nervosa; OCD; panic disorder; selective mutism
What kind of drug interactions may SSRIs produce?	Inhibition of cytochrome P-450 enzymes
Do SSRIs cause sexual dysfunction?	Yes, they can cause anorgasmia.
Do SSRIs cause cardiac arrhythmias?	No, they do not, in contrast to TCAs.
What are the adverse effects of SSRIs?	Sexual dysfunction; agitation; anxiety; seizures (with overdose); nausea; vomiting; diarrhea; sedation
Which SSRI is also FDA approved for social anxiety disorder (SAD), generalized anxiety disorder (GAD), and posttraumatic stress disorder (PTSD)?	Paroxetine
Which SSRIs cause the least amount of drug-drug interactions?	Citalopram; escitalopram; sertraline

AGENTS FOR MANIC-DEPRESSION

Manic-depression is also known as what?	Bipolar disorder
What is the traditional drug of choice for treating manic-depression?	Lithium
When is lithium used in the treatment of manic-depression (what phases of the disease)?	Prevention; treatment of manic episodes
Does lithium have a narrow or wide therapeutic window?	Narrow. Therapeutic levels range from 0.6 to 1.2 mEq/L and toxicity is seen at 1.5 mEq/L (and at 0.8 mEq/L in elderly patients).
Lithium is eliminated renally in a similar fashion to which other salt?	Sodium
Is lithium toxicity exacerbated by low or high sodium plasma levels?	Low sodium levels

What is the mechanism of action of lithium?

Unknown; may decrease cAMP levels thereby decreasing its function as a second messenger; may inhibit dephosphorylation of IP_3 to IP_2 and IP_2 to IP thereby interfering with the recycling of inositol

What are the adverse effects of lithium?

Acne; seizures; visual disturbances; edema; ataxia; drug-induced nephrogenic diabetes insipidus; hypothyroidism; tremors

How does lithium cause drug-induced nephrogenic diabetes insipidus?

Uncoupling of the vasopressin V_2 receptor in the kidney

Which diuretic is usually used to treat nephrogenic diabetes insipidus?

Thiazide diuretics

Which drug is used to treat lithium-induced nephrogenic diabetes insipidus?

Amiloride (thiazide diuretics cause increased reabsorption of lithium which may lead to lithium toxicity)

How does lithium cause hypothyroidism?

Inhibition of 5′-deiodinase

What is 5′-deiodinase responsible for?

Converting thyroxine (T4) to triiodothyronine (T3)

What is the name of the cardiac anomaly that may be found in neonates born to mothers using lithium?

Ebstein anomaly

What characterizes Ebstein anomaly?

Malformation of the tricuspid valve leaflets (partly attached to the fibrous tricuspid valve annulus; partly attached to the right ventricular endocardium; inferior displacement of the tricuspid leaflets)

What other medications (mood stabilizers) may be used in the treatment of manic-depression?

Carbamazepine; valproic acid; benzodiazepines; gabapentin; topiramate

Why are antidepressant agents not used to treat the depression phase of manic-depression?

May cause patients to enter into the manic phase

ANTIPSYCHOTIC AGENTS

According to the dopamine (DA) hypothesis of schizophrenia, do symptoms arise due to an excess or a lack of DA in the CNS?

An excess of DA

What characterizes the positive symptoms of schizophrenia?

Hallucinations; delusions; thought disorders

What characterizes the negative symptoms of schizophrenia?

Speech disorders; flat affect; amotivation; social withdrawal

What is the mechanism of action of "typical" antipsychotic agents?

Inhibition of D_2 receptors in the mesolimbic system of the brain

What is the mechanism of action of "atypical" antipsychotic agents?

Inhibition of $5\text{-}HT_2$ receptors (D_2 receptors are still involved to some extent)

Give examples of typical antipsychotics:

Haloperidol; chlorpromazine; thioridazine; fluphenazine; pimozide

Give examples of atypical antipsychotics:

Clozapine; risperidone; aripiprazole; olanzapine; ziprasidone; quetiapine

Name two typical antipsychotics commonly used in the treatment of Tourette syndrome:

1. Haloperidol
2. Pimozide

What are extrapyramidal symptoms (EPS)?

Parkinsonian-like symptoms (dystonia, rigidity, tremor, and bradykinesia); akathisia; tardive dyskinesia (TD)

What is akathisia?

Motor restlessness

What is tardive dyskinesia (TD)?

Inappropriate movements of the tongue, neck, trunk, and limbs (associated with long-term use of DA antagonists)

What is the mechanism of antipsychotic-induced TD?

Long-term DA receptor inhibition leads to an upregulation and supersensitivity of DA receptors, thereby leading to DA overstimulation, especially when the antipsychotic has been discontinued.

Which antipsychotics are more likely to cause EPS?

High potency typical antipsychotics such as haloperidol and fluphenazine secondary to their weak anticholinergic activity

Why do thioridazine and chlorpromazine have a lower EPS potential?

They have high anticholinergic activity.

What medications are used to treat antipsychotic-induced EPS?

Benztropine; amantadine; diphenhydramine (due to its anticholinergic action)

How do antipsychotics cause parkinsonian-like symptoms?

Inhibition of DA receptors in the nigrostriatal pathway

How do antipsychotics cause orthostatic hypotension?

Inhibition of α-adrenergic receptors in the vasculature

How do antipsychotics cause prolactinemia?

Inhibition of DA receptors in the anterior pituitary

Which two antipsychotics possess the highest antimuscarinic activity?

1. Chlorpromazine
2. Thioridazine

Characterize the antimuscarinic activity of chlorpromazine and thioridazine:

Xerostomia; blurred vision; confusion; constipation; urinary retention

What is xerostomia?

Dry mouth

Which antipsychotic agents are more effective at treating negative symptoms?

Atypical antipsychotics

Which phenothiazine antipsychotic is also used to treat intractable hiccups?

Chlorpromazine

Which phenothiazine antipsychotic may cause priapism, agranulocytosis, blue-gray discoloration of the skin, and lower seizure threshold?

Thioridazine

Which two typical antipsychotics can be formulated as depot intramuscular injections that may last up to 3 weeks?

1. Haloperidol
2. Fluphenazine

Which atypical antipsychotic is usually reserved as a third-line agent to treat schizophrenic patients refractory to traditional therapy?

Clozapine

What is the major dose-limiting side effect of clozapine?

Agranulocytosis

How are patients receiving clozapine therapy monitored?	WBCs obtained at baseline and weekly for the first 6 months of therapy, every other week for the second 6 months, and monthly thereafter
What adverse effect is more common with clozapine, agranulocytosis, or seizures?	Seizures (occur in 10% of patients, whereas agranulocytosis occurs in 1%-2% of patients)
Why is gynecomastia a common adverse effect of risperidone?	Risperidone induces prolactinemia (only atypical antipsychotic that increases prolactin levels significantly)
What is a potential life-threatening adverse effect of antipsychotic medications?	Neuroleptic malignant syndrome (NMS)
What characterizes NMS?	Hyperthermia; rigidity; altered mental status; cardiovascular instability
What is the treatment for NMS?	Dantrolene + bromocriptine (DA agonist)
What are the additional adverse effects of olanzapine?	Weight gain; hyperglycemia; sialorrhea
What are the additional adverse effects of quetiapine?	Hypercholesterolemia; hypertriglyceridemia; weight gain; hepatotoxicity
What is the mechanism of action of aripiprazole?	Antagonist at $5\text{-}HT_{2A}$ receptors; partial agonist at D_2 and $5\text{-}HT_{1A}$ receptors
What are the additional adverse effects of aripiprazole?	Weight gain; rash; sialorrhea; hepatotoxicity
Which antipsychotic has the highest incidence of sialorrhea?	Clozapine (31%-48%)

AGENTS FOR PARKINSON DISEASE

What are the signs of Parkinson disease (PD)?	Bradykinesia; muscular rigidity; tremors; gait abnormalities; postural instability
What neurotransmitter pathway is affected in PD?	Dopaminergic pathway (inhibitory neurons) in the substantia nigra and corpus striatum (neurotransmitter ratio shifts toward decreased DA and increased acetylcholine [ACh])

What does increased levels of DA in the tuberoinfundibular tract lead to?	Decreased prolactin levels
What does increased levels of DA in the CTZ lead to?	Increased emesis
What does increased levels of DA in the mesolimbic-mesocortical tracts lead to?	Increased psychomotor activity; psychosis; schizophrenia; increased reinforcement
Which DA receptor subtype is implicated in PD?	D_2 receptor subtype (inhibitory receptor subtype that decreases cyclic adenosine monophosphate [cAMP] levels in the corpus striatum)
Given the abnormal DA/ACh shift in the striatum, give two pharmacologic strategies in the treatment of PD:	1. Medications that will increase DA levels 2. Medications that will decrease ACh levels
Do anti-Parkinson medications effect pathology, symptoms, or both?	Symptoms
Name two antimuscarinic medications that are used in the treatment of PD:	1. Benztropine 2. Trihexyphenidyl
Is benztropine more or less lipid soluble than atropine?	More lipid soluble (therefore, greater CNS penetration)
Which characteristic of PD is not affected by anticholinergics?	Bradykinesia
Is benztropine useful in the treatment of tardive dyskinesia?	No, it may actually exacerbate tardive dyskinesia.
What are the adverse effects of benztropine and trihexyphenidyl?	Xerostomia; blurred vision; constipation; urinary retention; sedation; mydriasis
How does amantadine work in the treatment of PD?	May inhibit reuptake of DA into presynaptic neurons; may increase DA release from presynaptic fibers
Amantadine is used to treat what condition other than PD?	Influenza A
What is the name of the dermatologic adverse effect caused by amantadine?	Livedo reticularis
What is livedo reticularis?	A network-patterned discoloration of the skin caused by dilation of capillaries and venules

Which characteristic of PD is not affected by amantadine?	Tremors
Which selective MAO$_B$ inhibitor is commonly used as first-line treatment for PD?	Selegiline
What is the mechanism of action of selegiline?	Inhibition of DA metabolism in presynaptic neurons located in the CNS via inhibition of MAO$_B$
What are the two active metabolites of selegiline?	1. Amphetamine 2. Methamphetamine
What are the main adverse effects of selegiline?	Cardiovascular stimulation (hypertension, tachycardia, palpitations; arrhythmias; angina)
Name two ergot derivatives that act as DA agonists in the nigrostriatal system:	1. Bromocriptine 2. Pergolide
Bromocriptine is used to treat what conditions other than PD?	Prolactin-secreting microadenomas; NMS; acromegaly; postpartum lactation
What are the adverse effects of bromocriptine?	Headache; dizziness; nausea; orthostatic hypotension; dyskinesia; hallucinations; confusion; psychosis
Name two nonergot DA agonists:	1. Pramipexole 2. Ropinirole
What are the adverse effects of the nonergot DA agonists?	Sedation; syncope; nausea; vomiting; hallucinations; dyskinesia
What is the mechanism of action of tolcapone and entacapone?	Inhibition of peripheral catechol-O-methyltransferase (COMT), thereby increasing CNS uptake of L-dopa
What reaction does COMT catalyze?	Conversion of L-dopa to 3-O-methyldopa (partial DA agonist) in peripheral tissues
What are the adverse effects of COMT inhibitors?	Orthostatic hypotension; headache; fatigue; nausea; diarrhea; anorexia; dyskinesia; muscle cramps; brown-orange urine discoloration; hallucinations; diaphoresis
Which of the COMT inhibitors is hepatotoxic?	Tolcapone

Are COMT inhibitors used as first-line therapy, adjunctive therapy, or both in the treatment of PD?

Adjunctive therapy (in combination with carbidopa/levodopa)

Are the nonergot DA agonists used as first-line therapy, adjunctive therapy, or both in the treatment of PD?

Both

What is the precursor of DA?

Levodopa (L-dopa)

What enzyme converts L-dopa to DA?

Dopa decarboxylase (DDC)

Does DA cross the BBB?

No

Does levodopa cross the BBB?

Yes, it does and is subsequently converted to DA by dopaminergic neurons in the substantia nigra.

Is levodopa effective in treating PD when all of the dopaminergic neurons in the substantia nigra have been destroyed?

No, since dopaminergic neurons in the substantia nigra are required to convert levodopa to DA.

What is the mechanism of action of carbidopa?

Inhibition of peripheral DDC, thereby increasing the amount of levodopa that is available to cross the BBB into the CNS. This allows for lower doses of levodopa needed, thereby decreasing levodopa adverse effects.

Does carbidopa cross the BBB?

No, it does not and therefore only inhibits peripheral DDC.

How does levodopa work in the treatment of PD?

Decreases symptoms of PD, such as rigidity, bradykinesia, and tremors

What is the "on-off" phenomenon?

Levodopa has such a short half-life (1-2 h) that plasma concentrations may decline rapidly causing the patient to experience sudden rigidity, bradykinesia, and tremors.

Which amino acids compete with levodopa for GI absorption?

Isoleucine; leucine

What are the adverse effects of levodopa?

Anorexia; nausea; vomiting; tachycardia; hypotension; discoloration of saliva and urine; mydriasis; hallucinations; dyskinesia; increased intraocular pressure; cardiac arrhythmias

Why should vitamin B$_6$ (pyridoxine) not be used in combination with levodopa?	Pyridoxine enhances peripheral metabolism of levodopa, thereby rendering the medication ineffective.

ANTICONVULSANT AGENTS

What are the two types of partial seizures?	1. Simple 2. Complex
What are the three types of general seizures?	1. Tonic-clonic 2. Absence 3. Myoclonic
What is another name for tonic-clonic seizures?	Grand mal seizures
What is another name for absence seizures?	Petit mal seizures
Does hypoventilation or hyperventilation lower the seizure threshold?	Hyperventilation (via alkalinization of blood pH)
What is the most common seizure type?	Tonic-clonic seizure
What type of seizure is associated with "febrile seizures"?	Tonic-clonic seizure
What type of seizure most commonly presents during childhood?	Absence seizure
What is status epilepticus?	Epileptic seizure lasting longer than 30 minutes or absence of full recovery of consciousness between seizures (can be life threatening)
In general, how do antiepileptic agents work?	Inhibit initiation of an abnormal electrical discharge from the focal area; prevent dissemination of abnormal electrical discharge to surrounding areas of the brain
What is the mechanism of action of phenytoin?	Inhibition of axonal sodium channels to produce membrane stabilization
Does phenytoin inhibit the axonal sodium channel in its activated or inactivated state?	Inactivated state

What antiarrhythmic class does phenytoin belong to?

Class Ib

What type of drug interactions can phenytoin produce?

Induces cytochrome P-450 metabolic enzymes; highly protein bound, therefore, can potentially displace other medications from plasma proteins

What are the adverse effects of phenytoin?

Diplopia; sedation; ataxia; gingival hyperplasia; acne; hirsutism; megaloblastic anemia (interferes with folate absorption); granulocytopenia; hypotension (IV); osteomalacia; drug-induced lupus; hyperglycemia; nystagmus; Stevens-Johnson syndrome; hepatotoxicity

Is phenytoin safe to use during pregnancy?

No, it causes fetal hydantoin syndrome characterized by cleft lip and palate.

What prodrug is hydrolyzed to phenytoin and is commonly given intravenously secondary to its superior water solubility versus phenytoin?

Fosphenytoin

Name two other medications that may cause gingival hyperplasia:

1. Cyclosporin A
2. Nifedipine

Which types of seizures does phenytoin treat?

Simple partial; complex partial; tonic-clonic; status epilepticus

What is the mechanism of action of carbamazepine?

Inhibition of axonal sodium channels to produce membrane stabilization

What type of drug interactions can carbamazepine produce?

Induces cytochrome P-450 metabolic enzymes; auto-induces its own metabolism

What conditions, other than epilepsy, can carbamazepine be used in?

Manic-depression; trigeminal neuralgia

What are the adverse effects of carbamazepine?

Diplopia; sedation; ataxia; osteomalacia; aplastic anemia; hyponatremia; Stevens-Johnson syndrome; alopecia; pancreatitis; hepatotoxicity; nystagmus

Is carbamazepine safe to use in pregnancy?

No, it causes neural tube defects and craniofacial abnormalities.

Which types of seizures does carbamazepine treat?

Simple partial; complex partial; tonic-clonic

What antiepileptic medication can cause alopecia?	Valproic acid (VPA)
What is the mechanism of action of VPA?	Inhibition of axonal sodium channels; inhibition of T-type calcium channels; inhibition of GABA transaminase
What type of drug interactions can VPA produce?	Inhibition of cytochrome P-450 enzymes
What conditions, other than epilepsy, can VPA be used in?	Manic-depression; migraine
What are the adverse effects of VPA?	Hepatotoxicity; pancreatitis; alopecia; nausea; vomiting; photosensitivity; sedation; diarrhea; abdominal pain; thrombocytopenia; rash; amenorrhea; dysmenorrhea; weight gain; tinnitus
Is VPA safe to use in pregnancy?	No, it causes neural tube defects.
Which types of seizures does VPA treat?	Simple partial; complex partial; tonic-clonic; absence; myoclonic
Which antiepileptic medication is used to treat partial and tonic-clonic seizures during pregnancy?	Phenobarbital
Which benzodiazepines are used in the treatment of status epilepticus?	Diazepam; lorazepam
Which benzodiazepine is used to treat myoclonic and absence seizures?	Clonazepam
Which antiepileptic medication is the drug of choice for treating absence seizures and its only FDA indication is for absence seizures?	Ethosuximide
What is the mechanism of action of ethosuximide?	Inhibition of T-type calcium channels in the thalamus
What are the adverse effects of ethosuximide?	EPS; nausea; vomiting; diarrhea; abdominal pain; fatigue; hirsutism; Stevens-Johnson syndrome; drug-induced lupus; hiccups
Which antiepileptics decrease the efficacy of oral contraceptives?	Phenytoin; carbamazepine

How do phenytoin and carbamazepine decrease the efficacy of oral contraceptives?	Induction of cytochrome P-450 enzymes
Overdose or abrupt withdrawal of antiepileptics may cause what adverse effect?	Seizures
Give examples of newer antiepileptic medications:	Gabapentin; pregabalin; lamotrigine; topiramate; tiagabine; vigabatrin; felbamate; levetiracetam
Name two antiepileptics that are considered free of drug-drug interactions:	1. Levetiracetam 2. Gabapentin
Which of the newer antiepileptics may inhibit carbonic anhydrase, thereby causing a metabolic acidosis?	Topiramate
What conditions, other than epilepsy, can topiramate be used in?	Migraine; manic-depression; neuropathic pain
What is the mechanism of action of topiramate?	Inhibition of glutamate (AMPA) receptors; increases GABA effects; blocks neuronal voltage-gated sodium channels
Which types of seizures does topiramate treat?	Simple partial; complex partial; seizures associated with Lennox-Gastaut syndrome
What are the adverse effects of topiramate?	Impaired cognition; word finding difficulty; sedation; weight loss; renal stones; metabolic acidosis
Which of the newer antiepileptics may cause Stevens-Johnson syndrome?	Lamotrigine
What is the mechanism of action of lamotrigine?	Inhibition of sodium channels; inhibition of glutamate receptors
Which types of seizures does lamotrigine treat?	Absence; simple partial; complex partial; seizures associated with Lennox-Gastaut syndrome
What are the adverse effects of lamotrigine?	Stevens-Johnson syndrome; sedation; headache; dizziness; ataxia; nausea; diplopia; amenorrhea; dysmenorrhea

What neurotransmitter is gabapentin structurally related to?	GABA
Does gabapentin bind to the GABA receptor?	No
What is the mechanism of action of gabapentin?	Unknown (may bind to voltage-gated calcium channels specifically possessing the α-2-δ-1 subunit)
Which types of seizures does gabapentin treat?	Simple partial; complex partial
What conditions, other than epilepsy, can gabapentin be used in?	Migraine; neuropathic pain; manic-depression; insomnia; chronic pain; social phobia
What are the adverse effects of gabapentin?	Sedation; ataxia; viral infection (in children); weight gain; diarrhea; nausea; vomiting

AGENTS FOR MIGRAINE

What antihypertensive medication is used in the prophylaxis of migraine headache?	Propranolol
Give examples of medications in the "triptan" drug class:	Sumatriptan; almotriptan; naratriptan; rizatriptan; zolmitriptan
What is the mechanism of action of sumatriptan?	5-HT$_{1D}$-receptor agonist which causes vasoconstriction in cranial arteries
Why should sumatriptan be used with caution in a patient with angina?	Can precipitate an anginal attack secondary to vasospasm of coronary arteries
How long after the first dose can a second dose of sumatriptan be given if migraine headache has not resolved?	Dose may be repeated once after 2 hours.
What is the mechanism of action of the ergot alkaloids?	Causes vasoconstriction of cranial arteries less selectively than "triptans" by acting as an agonist at various 5-HT receptors throughout the body

Give examples of ergot alkaloids:	Ergotamine; ergonovine
What are some common side effects of ergotamine?	Nausea; vomiting; diarrhea; chest pain; toxic levels can cause gangrene
Why is ergotamine sometimes given with caffeine?	Caffeine increases gut absorption of ergotamine.
Are opioid analgesics usually effective against migraine headache?	No

CLINICAL VIGNETTES

A 39-year-old man is unsatisfied with the results he is seeing from his current antidepressant therapy. He decides to stop taking the medication and to start seeing a new psychiatrist. To avoid repeating the same therapy he does not reveal that he was previously treated for his major depressive disorder. The new psychiatrist prescribes a first-line SSRI to treat the patient. Shortly after taking the SSRI, the patient becomes tachycardic, diaphoretic, and experiences myoclonic twitches. He develops a generalized tonic-clonic seizure shortly after admission to the emergency room. What class of medication was the patient most likely taking previously?

This patient was most likely taking a monoamine oxidase inhibitor (MAOI) prior to his arrival at his new psychiatrist. Results may not be seen for up to a month after initiation of treatment with an MAOI, leading to patient dissatisfaction and the belief that the medication is not effective. Should the MAOI therapy be discontinued, adequate time should be allowed for complete clearance of the drug before alternate therapy is initiated. SSRIs are particularly dangerous when combined with MAOIs because of their risk for causing serotonin syndrome, which this patient has developed.

An 80-year-old man has come to a cocktail party celebrating the end-of-the-year holidays. At the party he enjoys some hors d'oeuvres including small sausages and cheeses. In a few minutes, however, he collapses and is rushed to the emergency room. There he is found to have a blood pressure of 200/98. His wife informs the physician that he only takes one antihypertensive medication. What medication does he most likely take, and how has it contributed to his current condition?

He has suffered a hypertensive crisis due to the combination of tyramine and MAOIs. Cured meats and aged cheeses, such as those consumed by the patient contain tyramine, which may displace norepinephrine from storage vesicles and cause a buildup of catecholamines, leading to extreme hypertension.

A 29-year-old man is undergoing abdominal surgery. Shortly after induction and successful intubation, the patient's peak airway pressures begin to rise. Bilateral auscultation confirms equal breath sounds, and stat chest x-ray reveals no pneumothorax. What intravenous anesthetic agent is most likely responsible for this development?

> Fentanyl, a synthetic high-potency opioid, is frequently used as a part of balanced anesthesia and can cause chest wall and laryngeal rigidity, interfering with mechanical ventilation. Low doses of opiates should be used to avoid this complication.

A 72-year-old woman with Parkinson disease is unable to move after sitting through a film at the movie theater with her family. What is the most likely therapy she is receiving for her disease, and why might the medication be responsible for her current situation? What fast-acting dopamine agonist would be appropriate for use in such a situation?

> The patient is most likely on levodopa therapy. Levodopa has a very short half-life leading to the "on-off" phenomenon frequently seen with its use. Patients may find they are suddenly unable to stand or walk and may require rescue therapy with a fast-acting dopamine agonist. Apomorphine is such an agent, and is useful in emergency situations such as that presented in the vignette. It does not require enzymatic conversion to an active product, and so works quickly—about 10 minutes after injection. Nausea and vomiting limit its use to rescue situations, as does dyskinesia and hypotension.

CHAPTER 6

Cardiovascular/Renal Agents

ANTIARRHYTHMIC (ANTIDYSRRHYTHMIC) AGENTS

Describe what happens during each of the following phases of the cardiac action potential for fast-response fibers:

Phase 0

Sodium ion channels open (inward) which leads to membrane depolarization.

Phase I

Sodium ion channels are inactivated; potassium ion channels (outward) are activated; chloride ion channels (inward) are activated.

Phase II

Plateau phase; slow influx of calcium ion balanced by outward potassium ion current (delayed rectifier current I_K)

Phase III

Repolarization phase; outward K^+ current increases and inward calcium ion current decreases

Phase IV

Membrane returns to resting potential.

FAST RESPONSE ACTION POTENTIALS

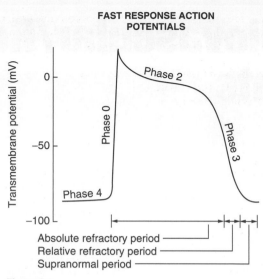

Figure 6.1

On what phase(s) of the cardiac action potential do amiodarone and sotalol work?	Phase 0 and phase III
On what phase(s) of the cardiac action potential do lidocaine, flecainide, and quinidine work?	Phase 0
On what phase(s) of the cardiac action potential do β-blockers work?	Phase II and phase IV
What is responsible for maintaining the electrochemical gradient at resting membrane potential?	Na^+/K^+-ATPase
What ion current is responsible for the depolarization of sinoatrial (SA) and atrioventricular (AV) nodal fibers?	Calcium ion (inward)
What ion current is responsible for the repolarization of SA and AV nodal fibers?	Potassium ion (outward)
How does phase IV of the action potential in slow-response fibers (SA and AV nodes) differ from that of fast-response fibers?	Slow-response fibers display automaticity (ability to depolarize spontaneously); rising phase IV slope of the action potential = pacemaker potential

What ion current is responsible for the "pacemaker current" (rising slope of phase IV) in slow-response fibers?

Sodium ion (inward); calcium ion (inward); potassium ion (outward)

The pacemaker of the heart has the fastest uprising phase IV slope; where is this pacemaker in nondiseased patients?

SA node

Where is the SA node located?

Right atrium

How do the effective refractory period (ERP) and relative refractory period (RRP) differ from each other?

No stimulus, no matter the strength, can elicit a response with fibers in the ERP, whereas a strong enough stimulus will elicit a response with fibers in the RRP.

What are the three states the voltage-gated Na^+ channel exists in?

1. Resting state
2. Open state
3. Inactivated state

What state(s) of the voltage-gated Na^+ channel is/are most susceptible to drugs?

Open state; inactivated state

What two types of gates does the voltage-gated Na^+ channel have?

1. M (activating)
2. H (inactivating)

Why is the rate of recovery from an action potential slower in ischemic tissue?

The cells are already partly depolarized at rest.

What class of antiarrhythmic agents has membrane stabilizing effects?

β-Blockers

Antiarrhythmic agents are grouped into four classes according to what classification system?

Vaughn-Williams classification

Give the general mechanism of action for each of the following antiarrhythmic drug classes:

Class I

Na^+ channel blockers

Class II

β-Blockers

Class III

K^+ channel blockers

Class IV

Ca^{++} channel blockers

Class I antiarrhythmics are further subdivided into what classes?

Ia; Ib; Ic

Give examples of antiarrhythmic drugs in class Ia:

Quinidine (antimalarial/antiprotozoal agent); procainamide; disopyramide

Give examples of antiarrhythmic drugs in class Ib:

Lidocaine; mexiletine; tocainide; phenytoin

Give examples of antiarrhythmic drugs in class Ic:

Encainide; flecainide; propafenone; moricizine

Give examples of antiarrhythmic drugs in class II:

Propranolol; esmolol; metoprolol

Give examples of antiarrhythmic drugs in class III:

Amiodarone; sotalol; ibutilide; dofetilide

Give examples of antiarrhythmic drugs in class IV:

Verapamil; diltiazem

Name three antiarrhythmic drugs that do not fit in the Vaughn-Williams classification system:

1. Digoxin
2. Adenosine
3. Magnesium

Magnesium is used to treat what specific type of arrhythmia?

Torsades de pointes (polymorphic ventricular tachycardia)

Adenosine is used to treat what types of arrhythmias?

Paroxysmal supraventricular tachycardia (PSVT), specifically narrow complex tachycardia or supraventricular tachycardia (SVT) with aberrancy; AV nodal arrhythmias (adenosine causes transient AV block). Note: synchronized cardioversion and *not* adenosine should be used on symptomatic patients or unstable tachycardia with pulses.

Where anatomically should the IV be placed to administer adenosine?

As close to the heart as possible, that is, the antecubital fossa since adenosine has an extremely short half-life. Adenosine rapid IV push should be followed immediately by a 5-10 cc (mL) flush of saline to facilitate its delivery to the heart.

What is the mechanism of action of adenosine?

Stimulates α_1-receptors which causes a decrease in cyclic adenosine monophosphate (cAMP) (via G_i-coupled second messenger system); increases K^+ efflux leading to increased hyperpolarization; increases refractory period in AV node

What are the adverse effects of adenosine?	Flushing; chest pain; dyspnea; hypotension
What two drugs can antagonize the effects of adenosine?	1. Theophylline 2. Caffeine
How is adenosine dosed?	6 mg initially by rapid IV push; if not effective within 1-2 minutes, give 12 mg repeat dose (follow each bolus of adenosine with normal saline flush). The 12 mg dose may be repeated once.
What is the most deadly ion that can be administered?	Potassium ion
What ECG changes are seen in hyperkalemia?	Flattened P waves; widened QRS complex; peaked T waves; sine waves; ventricular fibrillation
What ECG changes are seen in hypokalemia?	Flattened or inverted T waves; U waves; ST-segment depression
What do class Ia antiarrhythmics do to each of the following?	
Action potential duration	Increase
ERP	Increase
Conduction velocity	Decrease
Phase IV slope	Decrease
What do class Ib antiarrhythmics do to each of the following?	
Action potential duration	Decrease
ERP	Little or no change
Conduction velocity	Decrease (primarily in ischemic tissue)
Phase IV slope	Decrease
What do class Ic antiarrhythmics do to each of the following?	
Action potential duration	Little or no change
ERP	Little or no change
Conduction velocity	Decrease
Phase IV slope	Decrease

Drugs that affect the strength of heart muscle contraction are referred to as what types of agents?	Inotropes (either positive or negative)
Drugs that affect the heart rate are referred to as what types of agents?	Chronotropes (either positive or negative)
Drugs that affect AV conduction velocity are referred to as what types of agents?	Dromotropes (either positive or negative)
QT interval prolongation, and therefore torsades de pointes, is more likely to occur with what two classes of antiarrhythmics?	1. Ia 2. III
Which class Ia antiarrhythmic also blocks α-adrenergic and muscarinic receptors, thereby potentially leading to increased heart rate and AV conduction?	Quinidine
What are the adverse effects of quinidine?	Tachycardia; proarrhythmic; increased digoxin levels via protein-binding displacement; nausea; vomiting; diarrhea; cinchonism
What is cinchonism?	Syndrome that may include tinnitus; high-frequency hearing loss; deafness; vertigo; blurred vision; diplopia; photophobia; headache; confusion; delirium
What are the adverse effects of procainamide?	Drug-induced lupus (25%-30% of patients); proarrhythmic; depression; psychosis; hallucination; nausea; vomiting; diarrhea; agranulocytosis; thrombocytopenia; hypotension
What drugs can cause drug-induced lupus?	Procainamide; isoniazid (INH); chlorpromazine; penicillamine; sulfasalazine; hydralazine; methyldopa; quinidine; phenytoin; minocycline; valproic acid; carbamazepine; chlorpromazine
Which class Ia antiarrhythmic can cause peripheral vasoconstriction?	Disopyramide

What are the adverse effects of disopyramide?	Anticholinergic adverse effects, such as urinary retention; dry mouth; dry eyes; blurred vision; constipation; sedation
True or False? Lidocaine is useful in the treatment of ventricular arrhythmias?	True
True or False? Lidocaine is useful in the treatment of atrial arrhythmias?	False
True or False? Lidocaine is useful in the treatment of AV junctional arrhythmias?	False
What are the adverse effects of lidocaine?	Proarrhythmic; sedation; agitation; confusion; paresthesias; seizures
What class Ib antiarrhythmic is structurally related to lidocaine?	Mexiletine
What class Ib antiarrhythmic can cause pulmonary fibrosis?	Tocainide
Propafenone, even though a class Ic antiarrhythmic, exhibits what other type of antiarrhythmic activity?	β-Adrenergic receptor blockade
What famous trial showed that encainide and flecainide increased sudden cardiac death in postmyocardial infarction (MI) patients with arrhythmias?	Cardiac Arrhythmia Suppression Trial (CAST)
Sotalol, even though a class III antiarrhythmic, exhibits what other type of antiarrhythmic activity?	β-Adrenergic receptor blockade
Even though this agent is labeled as a Vaughn-Williams class III antiarrhythmic, it displays class I, II, III, and IV antiarrhythmic activity.	Amiodarone
What is the half-life of amiodarone?	40 to 60 days

What are the adverse effects of amiodarone?

Pulmonary fibrosis; tremor; ataxia; dizziness; hyperthyroidism; hypothyroidism; hepatotoxicity; photosensitivity; blue skin discoloration; neuropathy; muscle weakness; proarrhythmic; corneal deposits; lipid abnormalities; hypotension; nausea; vomiting; congestive heart failure (CHF); optic neuritis; pneumonitis; abnormal taste; abnormal smell; syndrome of inappropriate secretion of antidiuretic hormone (SIADH)

How should patients on amiodarone therapy be monitored?

ECG; thyroid function tests (TFTs); pulmonary function tests (PFTs); liver function tests (LFTs); electrolytes; ophthalmology examinations

Verapamil should not be given in what types of arrhythmias?

Wolff-Parkinson-White (WPW) syndrome; ventricular tachycardia

What are the adverse effects of verapamil?

Drug interactions; constipation; hypotension; AV block; CHF; dizziness; flushing

Digoxin is used to control ventricular rate in what types of arrhythmias?

Atrial fibrillation; atrial flutter

Digoxin-induced arrhythmias are treated by what drugs?

Lidocaine; phenytoin

Digoxin does what to each of the following?

    Strength of heart muscle contraction

Increases (positive inotrope)

    Heart rate

Decreases (negative chronotrope)

    AV conduction velocity

Decreases (negative dromotrope)

What does QTc stand for?

Corrected QT interval

How is QTc calculated?

(QT)/(square root of R to R interval)

Why must the QT interval be corrected?

The QT interval is dependent on heart rate, so higher heart rates will display shorter QT intervals on ECG. It is corrected to remove the variable of the heart rate.

What is the normal value for QTc?

Less than 440 milliseconds

What does a long QT interval put a patient at risk for? | Torsades de pointes, a ventricular arrhythmia that can degenerate into ventricular fibrillation

CONGESTIVE HEART FAILURE AGENTS

What is the cardiac output equation? | Cardiac output (CO) = heart rate (HR) × stroke volume (SV)

What is normal CO? | 5 L/min

What is the most common cause of right-sided heart failure? | Left-sided heart failure

Name three compensatory physiologic responses seen in congestive heart failure (CHF):
1. Fluid retention
2. Increased sympathetic drive
3. Hypertrophy of cardiac muscle

Define preload: | The pressure stretching the ventricular walls at the onset of ventricular contraction; related to left ventricular end-diastolic volume/pressure

Define afterload: | The load or force developed by the ventricle during systole

What drugs are used to decrease preload? | Diuretics; vasodilators; angiotensin-converting enzyme inhibitors (ACEIs); angiotensin II receptor blockers (ARBs); nitrates

What drugs are used to decrease afterload? | Vasodilators; ACEIs; ARBs; hydralazine

What drugs are used to increase contractility? | Digoxin; phosphodiesterase inhibitors (amrinone and milrinone); β-adrenoceptor agonists

What is the mechanism of action of digoxin? | Inhibition of the Na^+/K^+-ATPase pump which leads to positive inotropic action (via increased intracellular sodium ions that exchanges with extracellular calcium ions; resulting increase in intracellular calcium ions leads to increased force of contraction)

What are the two digitalis glycosides?
1. Digoxin
2. Digitoxin

What are the adverse effects of digoxin?
Arrhythmias; nausea; vomiting; anorexia; headache; confusion; blurred vision; visual disturbances, such as yellow halos around light sources

What electrolyte disturbances predispose to digoxin toxicity?
Hypokalemia; hypomagnesemia; hypercalcemia

Digoxin can cause what types of arrhythmias?
Supraventricular tachycardias; AV nodal tachycardias; AV block; ventricular tachycardias; ventricular fibrillation; complete heart block

Can digoxin be used in WPW syndrome?
No. Since digoxin slows conduction through the AV node, the accessory pathway present in WPW is left unopposed, leading to supraventricular tachycardias and atrial arrhythmias.

How is digoxin toxicity treated?
Correction of electrolyte disturbances; antiarrhythmics; anti-digoxin Fab antibody (Digibind)

What drugs can increase digoxin concentrations?
Quinidine; amiodarone; erythromycin; verapamil

What drugs can decrease digoxin concentrations?
Loop diuretics; thiazide diuretics; corticosteroids

Does digoxin therapy in CHF lead to prolonged survival?
No. It is of symptomatic benefit only, improving quality, but not necessarily duration of life.

What classes of medications have been shown to increase survival in CHF patients?
ACEs/ARBs; β-blockers

How does dobutamine work in CHF?
β-Adrenergic agonist (sympathomimetic that binds to β_1-adrenoceptors) that increases force of contraction and vasodilation via increased cAMP

How do amrinone and milrinone work in CHF?
Inhibits phosphodiesterase (PDE) thereby increasing cAMP levels; increased cAMP leads to increased intracellular calcium; increased intracellular calcium leads to increased force of contraction; increased cAMP also leads to increased vasodilation

What are the side effects of the PDEIs? | Milrinone may actually decrease survival in CHF; amrinone may cause thrombocytopenia.

How do diuretics work in CHF? | Decrease in intravascular volume thereby decrease in preload; reduce pulmonary and peripheral edema often seen in CHF patients

How can increased sympathetic activity in CHF be counteracted? | β-Blockers

What two β-blockers have specific indications for the treatment of CHF? | 1. Metoprolol
2. Carvedilol (mixed α-/β-blocker)

What is the mechanism of action of nesiritide? | Recombinant B-type natriuretic peptide that binds to guanylate cyclase receptors on vascular smooth muscle and endothelial cells, thereby increasing cyclic guanosine monophosphate (cGMP) levels; increased cGMP leads to increased relaxation of vascular smooth muscle

How do ACEIs work in CHF? | Inhibition of angiotensin-II (AT-II) production thereby decreasing total peripheral resistance (TPR) and thus afterload; prevents left ventricular remodeling

ANTIANGINAL AGENTS

Define angina pectoris: | Chest pain resulting from a myocardial oxygen demand that is not met by adequate oxygen supply; seen in patient with myocardial ischemia

What type of angina is caused by spontaneous coronary vasospasm? | Prinzmetal (variant) angina

What type of angina is caused by atherosclerosis of coronary vessels and is precipitated by exertion? | Classic angina

What type of angina can be acute in onset and is caused by platelet aggregation? | Unstable angina

What two mechanistic strategies are used in the treatment of angina?	1. Increase oxygen supply to the myocardium 2. Decrease myocardial oxygen demand
What types of drugs can increase oxygen supply?	Nitrates; calcium channel blockers (CCBs)
What types of drugs can decrease oxygen demand?	Nitrates; CCBs; β-blockers
What is the drug of choice for immediate relief of anginal symptoms?	Sublingual nitroglycerin (NTG)
What is the mechanism of action of nitrates?	Nitrates form nitrites; nitrites form nitric oxide (NO); NO activates guanylyl cyclase to increase cGMP; increased cGMP leads to increased relaxation of vascular smooth muscle
How does cGMP lead to relaxation of vascular smooth muscle?	Causes dephosphorylation of myosin light chains
How do nitrates increase oxygen supply?	Dilation of coronary vessels which leads to increased blood supply
How do nitrates decrease oxygen demand?	Dilation of large veins which leads to preload reduction; decreased preload reduces the amount of work done by the heart; decreased amount of work results in decreased myocardial oxygen requirement
What are the adverse effects of nitrates?	Headache; hypotension; reflex tachycardia; facial flushing; methemoglobinemia
Why must patients have at least a 10- to 12-hour "nitrate-free" interval every day?	Tolerance (tachyphylaxis) develops to nitrates if given on a continuous (around-the-clock) basis
Nitrates are contraindicated in patients taking any of what three medications?	1. Sildenafil 2. Vardenafil 3. Tadalafil
Methemoglobin formation, specifically by amyl nitrite, can be used to treat what type of poisoning?	Cyanide
What are the common formulations of nitrates?	NTG; isosorbide mononitrate; isosorbide dinitrate

What is the time to peak effect of sublingual NTG?	2 minutes
What is the dosing frequency of sublingual NTG during an anginal episode?	Every 5 minutes for a maximum of three doses
How do β-blockers work in the treatment of angina?	Inhibition of β_1-adrenoceptors which leads to decreased CO, HR, and force of contraction, thereby reducing the workload of the heart and oxygen demand
Do β-blockers increase oxygen supply?	No
For each of the following CCBs, state whether their primary effects are on the myocardium or peripheral vasculature:	
Verapamil	Myocardium (greater negative inotropic effects)
Dihydropyridines (DHP; nifedipine, amlodipine, felodipine, isradipine, nicardipine)	Peripheral vasculature (more potent vasodilators)
Diltiazem	Myocardium
How do CCBs work in the treatment of angina?	Block vascular L-type calcium channels which leads to decreased heart contractility and increased vasodilation

ANTIHYPERTENSIVE AGENTS

According to JNC 7 guidelines, please define the following:	
Normal blood pressure	<120/80 mm Hg
Prehypertension	120 to 139/80 to 89 mm Hg
Stage I hypertension	140 to 159/90 to 99 mm Hg
Stage II hypertension	≥160/100 mm Hg
What is the goal blood pressure (BP) in patients *without* diabetes mellitus (DM) or chronic kidney disease?	<140/90 mm Hg
What is the goal BP in patients *with* DM or chronic kidney disease?	<130/80 mm Hg

Define essential hypertension (HTN):	HTN of unknown etiology, that is, primary hypertension
True or False? The majority of HTN cases are essential.	True
What is the BP equation?	Blood pressure (BP) = cardiac output (CO) × total peripheral resistance (TPR)
What is responsible for moment-to-moment changes in BP?	Baroreceptor reflexes (autonomic nervous system)
Where are the baroreceptors that are sensitive to the moment-to-moment changes in BP located?	Aortic arch; carotid sinuses
What organ is responsible for the long- term control of BP?	Kidney
The kidney responds to reduced BP by releasing what peptidase?	Renin
Renin is responsible for what enzymatic reaction?	Conversion of angiotensinogen to angiotensin-I (AT-I)
What enzyme is responsible for converting AT-I to AT-II?	Angiotensin-converting enzyme (ACE)
Where is ACE found?	In the lungs
What function does AT-II have with regard to BP regulation?	Vasoconstriction (increases TPR thereby increases BP); stimulation of aldosterone release
Where is aldosterone synthesized?	Zona glomerulosa of the adrenal cortex
What function does aldosterone have with regard to BP regulation?	Increases reabsorption of sodium ion in exchange for potassium ion; water osmotically follows sodium ion, therefore, aldosterone leads to salt and water retention thereby increasing BP
What is the name of the most common thiazide diuretic used in the treatment of HTN?	Hydrochlorothiazide (HCTZ)
What are the immediate/acute effects of thiazide diuretics?	Increased sodium, chloride, and water excretion which leads to decreased blood volume
What are the chronic effects of thiazide diuretics?	Decreased TPR

What is the site of action of thiazide diuretics?

Distal convoluted tubule of nephron

What transporter (in the distal convoluted tubule) is inhibited by thiazide diuretics?

Na^+/Cl^- transporter

Give examples of thiazide diuretics:

HCTZ; chlorothiazide; chlorthalidone

Thiazide diuretics may be ineffective in patients with creatinine clearances of less than what?

50 mL/min

With regard to *blood* concentrations, state whether each of the following electrolytes will be increased or decreased in patients on thiazide diuretic therapy:

    Calcium

Increased

    Magnesium

Decreased

    Potassium

Decreased

    Sodium

Decreased

With regard to increased renal calcium reabsorption, what are thiazide diuretics sometimes used for?

Treatment of calcium stones in the urine

What are the adverse effects of HCTZ?

Hypercalcemia; hypokalemia; hypomagnesemia; hyperglycemia; hyperuricemia; pancreatitis; metabolic alkalosis; Stevens-Johnson syndrome; hyperlipidemia

Patients allergic to what class of antimicrobials may also be sensitive to thiazide diuretics?

Sulfonamides

What is the site of action of loop diuretics?

Loop of Henle (thick ascending limb)

Give examples of loop diuretics:

Furosemide; bumetanide; ethacrynic acid; torsemide

Which loop diuretic can be given safely to patients with allergy to sulfonamide antimicrobials?

Ethacrynic acid

What transporter (in the thick ascending loop of Henle) is inhibited by loop diuretics?

$Na^+/K^+/2Cl^-$ transporter

True or False? Loop diuretics increase calcium excretion.

True

What are the adverse effects of loop diuretics?

Hypersensitivity; hypocalcemia; hypokalemia; hypomagnesemia; metabolic alkalosis; hyperuricemia; ototoxicity

Which loop diuretic is the most ototoxic?

Ethacrynic acid

Which renal tubular segment is responsible for the majority of sodium reabsorption?

Proximal convoluted tubule (>60%)

What is the mechanism of action of mannitol?

Acts as an osmotic diuretic, thereby drawing water via increased osmolality, into the proximal convoluted tubule, loop of Henle (thin descending limb), and the collecting ducts

What is mannitol used for?

Decreases intraocular and intracranial pressure; prevents anuria in hemolysis and rhabdomyolysis

Give two examples of carbonic anhydrase inhibitors (CAIs):

1. Acetazolamide
2. Dorzolamide

What is the mechanism of action of CAIs?

Increased excretion of sodium and bicarbonate

What metabolic disturbance may be caused by CAIs?

Metabolic acidosis

What are CAIs used for?

Altitude sickness (decreases cerebral and pulmonary edema); glaucoma (decreases aqueous humor formation thereby decreasing intraocular pressure); metabolic alkalosis; to enhance renal excretion of acidic drugs

Name three potassium-sparing diuretics:

1. Spironolactone
2. Triamterene
3. Amiloride

What is the mechanism of action of spironolactone?

Aldosterone receptor antagonist

Where in the kidney is the aldosterone receptor found?

Basolateral membrane of the principal cell in the collecting duct

Where in the kidney does triamterene and amiloride work?

Sodium ion channel on the luminal side of the principal cell in the collecting duct

What are the adverse effects of spironolactone?

Hyperkalemia; metabolic acidosis; gynecomastia

Triamterene is often used in combination with what other diuretic?

HCTZ

Spironolactone is used to treat what conditions?

HTN; CHF; ascites

Amiloride is used to treat what conditions?

HTN; CHF; lithium-induced diabetes insipidus

With regard to BP = CO × TPR, how do β-blockers lower BP?

Decrease CO

What is the prototype β-blocker?

Propranolol

Is propranolol cardioselective?

No

Because of their cardioselectivity, what two β-blockers have gained the most widespread use?

1. Metoprolol
2. Atenolol

Patients with what specific disease states should not receive nonselective β-antagonists?

Asthma (increased risk of bronchospasm); diabetes; peripheral vascular disease

What action do β-blockers have on the kidneys?

They decrease renin release by preventing stimulation of renin release by catecholamines and also likely by direct depression of the renin-angiotensin-aldosterone system.

What are the adverse effects of β-blockers?

Hypotension; lipid abnormalities; rebound HTN with abrupt withdrawal; fatigue; insomnia; sexual dysfunction; hallucinations; depression; hyperglycemia

Which β-blocker has the shortest half-life?

Esmolol (9 min), therefore esmolol is usually administered as a continuous drip.

With regard to BP = CO × TPR, how do ACE inhibitors decrease BP?

Decrease TPR

In addition to conversion of AT-I to AT-II, what other reaction does ACE catalyze?

The breakdown of bradykinin. ACE is also known as kininase.

What action does bradykinin have on vascular smooth muscle?

Vasodilation

Increased bradykinin levels may lead to what adverse reaction experienced by patients who take ACE inhibitors?

Dry cough

How do ACE inhibitors decrease sodium and water retention?

Decreased levels of AT-II leads to decreased levels of aldosterone and therefore reduced sodium and water retention.

What are the adverse effects of ACE inhibitors?

Hypotension; dry cough; hyperkalemia; angioedema; fever; altered taste

Give examples of ACE inhibitors:

Benazepril; captopril; enalapril; fosinopril; lisinopril; quinapril; ramipril

Give two contraindications for ACE inhibitor therapy:

1. Pregnancy (teratogenic)
2. Bilateral renal artery stenosis

What is the mechanism of action of losartan?

AT-II receptor blocker

Give examples of ARBs:

Candesartan; eprosartan; irbesartan; losartan; olmesartan; telmisartan; valsartan

Which specific receptor type do ARBs antagonize?

AT-II type 1 receptor

Do ARBs cause dry cough?

No (ARBs do not inhibit the breakdown of bradykinin)

Is there a pregnancy contraindication for ARBs?

Yes, they are pregnancy category C for the first trimester and category D for the second and third trimester.

How do CCBs work in the treatment of HTN?

Block vascular L-type calcium channels which leads to decreased heart contractility and increased vasodilation of coronary and peripheral vasculature

What are the adverse effects of the DHP CCBs?

Peripheral edema; hypotension; reflex tachycardia; headache; flushing; gingival hyperplasia

What are the adverse effects of verapamil?	Drug-drug interactions; constipation; AV block; headache
What action do CCBs have on the kidney?	Natriuretic activity
Which CCB is used in subarachnoid hemorrhages to prevent vasospasm?	Nimodipine
Give an example of a T-type CCB used in the treatment of absence seizures:	Ethosuximide
Name three α_1-adrenergic antagonists used in the treatment of HTN:	1. Doxazosin 2. Prazosin 3. Terazosin
How do α_1-adrenergic antagonists decrease BP?	Antagonize α_1-receptors in vascular smooth muscle, thereby causing vasodilation and reduced TPR
What are the two main adverse effects of α_1-antagonists?	1. First dose syncope 2. Reflex tachycardia
What class of drugs can be used to block the reflex tachycardia caused by α_1-antagonists?	β-Blockers
α_1-Adrenergic antagonists are most commonly used for what condition other than hypertension?	Benign prostatic hyperplasia (BPH)
How does clonidine work as an antihypertensive?	Central α_2-adrenergic agonist (decreases sympathetic outflow from the CNS, producing a decrease in TPR, HR, and BP)
Why are diuretics often given to patients on clonidine therapy?	Clonidine causes sodium and water retention.
Other than HTN, what is clonidine used for?	Nicotine withdrawal; heroin withdrawal; alcohol dependence; migraine prophylaxis; severe pain; clozapine-induced sialorrhea
What are the adverse effects of clonidine?	Bradycardia; sedation; dry mouth; rebound HTN with abrupt withdrawal (must taper down dose when discontinuing therapy); edema

Can clonidine be used in patients with renal dysfunction?

Yes, because renal blood flow and glomerular filtration rate are not compromised with clonidine therapy.

α-Methyldopa is converted to what active metabolite?

Methylnorepinephrine

What is the mechanism of action of α-methyldopa?

Central α_2-adrenergic agonist

Can α-methyldopa be used in patients with renal dysfunction?

Yes

Is α-methyldopa contraindicated in pregnancy?

No, it is one of the antihypertensive drugs of choice in pregnant women.

What are the adverse effects of α-methyldopa?

Sedation; hemolytic anemia; drug-induced lupus; edema; bradycardia; dry mouth

What arterial vasodilator decreases TPR, often requires a β-blocker to counteract the subsequent reflex tachycardia, and may cause drug-induced lupus?

Hydralazine

What class of drugs are used to counteract the fluid retention caused by hydralazine?

Diuretics

What are the adverse effects of hydralazine?

Reflex tachycardia; fluid retention; drug-induced lupus; headache; flushing

What enzyme is responsible for the metabolism of hydralazine?

N-acetyltransferase

What is the mechanism of action of minoxidil?

Opens potassium channels which leads to membrane hyperpolarization and subsequent arterial vasodilation

Minoxidil is a prodrug that is activated by what mechanism?

Sulfation

What is a common side effect of minoxidil?

Hypertrichosis (used in the treatment of alopecia)

What drug is a direct acting vasodilator, used in hypertensive emergencies, and can also be used to prevent hypoglycemia in patients with insulinoma?

Diazoxide

How does diazoxide work to prevent hypoglycemia in patients with insulinoma?

It decreases insulin release.

What drug is used during hypertensive emergencies, acts via increasing cGMP through NO mechanisms, and forms thiocyanate and cyanide metabolites?

Sodium nitroprusside

What class of antihypertensives may help prevent left ventricular remodeling seen in patients with CHF?

ACE inhibitors

What class of antihypertensives may improve patients' lipid profiles?

α_1-Adrenergic antagonists

What two classes of antihypertensives may protect renal function in patients with DM?

ACE inhibitors and ARBs by decreasing microalbuminuria

ANTIHYPERLIPIDEMIC AGENTS

What is the mechanism of action of the "statin" class of antihyperlipidemics?

Inhibition of hydroxymethylglutaryl coenzyme A (HMG-CoA) reductase (rate-limiting step of cholesterol biosynthesis), thereby inhibiting the intracellular supply of cholesterol; increases number of cell surface low-density lipoproteins (LDL) receptors which further reduces plasma cholesterol levels via increased metabolism

How do statins affect the lipid profile?

Mainly reduces LDL; moderate reduction of triglycerides (TGs); moderate elevation of high-density lipoproteins (HDL)

Give examples of medications in the statin drug class:

Atorvastatin; rosuvastatin; simvastatin; pravastatin; lovastatin; fluvastatin

What are the adverse effects of statin drugs?

Increased liver function tests (LFTs); dose-dependent rhabdomyolysis, myalgia, and myopathy; diarrhea; drug-induced lupus; drug-drug interactions; contraindicated in pregnancy (category X)

What laboratory tests should be used to monitor for statin toxicity?	LFTs; creatine phosphokinase (CPK)
What is the most potent antihyperlipidemic agent to elevate high-density lipoprotein (HDL)?	Niacin
Niacin is also known as what?	Vitamin B_3; nicotinic acid
What is the mechanism of action of niacin?	High-dose niacin inhibits very low-density lipoprotein (VLDL) and apoprotein synthesis in hepatocytes; increases tissue plasminogen activator (tPA); decreases fibrinogen
How does niacin affect the lipid profile?	Elevation of HDL; reduction of LDL; reduction of VLDL; reduction of TGs
What are the adverse effects of niacin?	Facial flushing; hyperuricemia; hyperglycemia; hepatotoxicity; pruritus; nausea; abdominal pain
How is facial flushing counteracted in patients on niacin therapy?	Pretreatment with aspirin to counteract the prostaglandin release
What new antihyperlipidemic agent works by inhibiting absorption of cholesterol at the brush border in the small intestine?	Ezetimibe
What are the adverse effects of ezetimibe?	Diarrhea; abdominal pain; headache; arthralgias
Which antihyperlipidemic drug class decreases VLDL, LDL, TGs and increases HDL by activating lipoprotein lipase?	Fibrates
Give examples of medications in the fibrate drug class:	Gemfibrozil; clofibrate; fenofibrate
What is the major effect that fibrates have on the lipid profile?	Reduction of TGs
What are the adverse effects of gemfibrozil?	Cholelithiasis; nausea; diarrhea; abdominal pain; myositis; hypokalemia; increased levels of warfarin and sulfonylureas via protein-binding displacement

What is the mechanism of action of bile acid sequestrants?

Anion exchange resins that bind bile acids/salts in the small intestine, thereby preventing their reabsorption; decreased bile acids results in increased plasma cholesterol uptake by hepatocytes to replenish bile acid levels, thereby decreasing plasma LDL levels

Give examples of bile acid sequestrants:

Cholestyramine; colestipol; colesevelam

What are the adverse effects of bile acid sequestrants?

Constipation; bloating; flatulence; nausea; impaired absorption of fat-soluble vitamins; impaired absorption of warfarin; digoxin; acetyl salicylic acid (ASA); tetracycline (TCN); thiazide diuretics

What over-the-counter medication, naturally found in certain fish, can decrease TG levels and be useful in the prevention of coronary heart disease (CHD)?

Omega-3 fatty acids

ANTICOAGULATION AGENTS

Where is prostacyclin made?

Vascular endothelial cells

Where is thromboxane A_2 made?

Platelets

Increased prostacyclin leads to an increase of what second messenger?

cAMP

cAMP does what to platelets?

Inhibits platelet activation and release of platelet aggregating factors

How does ASA work as a platelet aggregation inhibitor?

Irreversible inhibition, via acetylation, of cyclooxygenase (COX) thereby reducing thromboxane A_2 levels

What two drugs inhibit platelet aggregation and platelet-fibrinogen interaction by blocking adenosine diphosphate (ADP) receptors?

1. Clopidogrel
2. Ticlopidine

What are the major adverse effects of ticlopidine?

Neutropenia; agranulocytosis; thrombotic thrombocytopenic purpura (TTP)

How should patients on ticlopidine therapy be monitored?	Complete blood count (CBC) with differential every 2 weeks for the first 3 months of therapy and as needed thereafter
How does dipyridamole work as a platelet aggregation inhibitor?	Inhibits phosphodiesterase (PDE) thereby increasing cAMP levels; cAMP potentiates prostacyclin and inhibits thromboxane A_2 synthesis
Dipyridamole is usually given in combination with what drug?	Aspirin
What are the two main systems that feed into the common pathway of the clotting cascade?	1. Intrinsic system 2. Extrinsic system
Activation of clotting factor VII to VIIa marks the beginning of which clotting system?	Extrinsic system
Activation of clotting factor XII to XIIa marks the beginning of which clotting system?	Intrinsic system
Activation of which clotting factor marks the beginning of the common pathway?	Activation of factor X to factor Xa
What is another name for factor II?	Prothrombin
What is another name for factor IIa?	Thrombin
What factor is also known as "Christmas factor"?	Factor IX
What factor is deficient in hemophilia A?	Factor VIII
What factor is deficient in hemophilia B?	Factor IX
How does heparin work as an anticoagulant?	Complexes with antithrombin-III to increase inactivation of clotting factors IIa, IXa, Xa, XIa, XIIa, and XIIIa
Which system of the clotting cascade is mainly affected by heparin?	Intrinsic system

Which laboratory test is used to monitor heparin therapy?	Partial thromboplastin time (PTT); therapeutic PTT levels are 1.5 to 2.5 times that of normal
How is heparin administered?	Intravenously (IV), subcutaneously (SQ)
Why is intramuscular administration of heparin contraindicated?	Hematoma formation
What are the therapeutic indications of heparin?	Prevention and treatment (by preventing expansion of the clot) of deep vein thrombosis (DVT) and pulmonary embolism (PE); used for anticoagulation during MI
What is the onset of action of heparin?	IV = immediate onset of action; SQ = 20 to 30 minutes
Does heparin cross the placental barrier?	No, therefore it is safe in pregnancy.
What are the adverse effects of heparin?	Bleeding; hypersensitivity; osteoporosis; heparin-induced thrombocytopenia (HIT)
Heparin undergoes what type of metabolism?	Hepatic; reticuloendothelial system
What drug is used to counteract heparin overdose?	Protamine sulfate
Roughly, how many units of heparin are neutralized by 1 mg of protamine sulfate?	100 units
What is the onset of action of protamine sulfate?	5 minutes
What paradoxical adverse effect can protamine cause at high doses?	Anticoagulation leading to hemorrhage
What is the mechanism of action of enoxaparin?	Low-molecular-weight heparin (LMWH) that has a higher ratio of antifactor Xa to antifactor IIa activity versus unfractionated heparin (UFH)
What is the half-life of LMWH?	Two to four times that of UFH
Does PTT need to be monitored in patients on LMWH therapy?	No

What synthetic pentasaccharide causes an antithrombin-III-mediated selective inhibition of factor Xa?	Fondaparinux
Which system of the clotting cascade is mainly affected by warfarin?	Extrinsic system
Which laboratory tests are used to monitor warfarin therapy?	Prothrombin time (PT); international normalized ratio (INR) → therapeutic INR levels are between 2 and 3
How does warfarin work as an anticoagulant?	Inhibits synthesis of vitamin-K-dependent clotting factors II, VII, IX, and X via inhibition of vitamin K epoxide reductase; also inhibits synthesis of protein C and protein S
What is the onset of action of warfarin?	36 to 72 hours (anticoagulant action)
How long after initiation of warfarin therapy is the full therapeutic effect seen?	5 to 7 days (antithrombotic action)
Acute alcohol intoxication does what to warfarin metabolism?	Inhibits warfarin metabolism, thereby increasing warfarin blood levels
Chronic alcohol use does what to warfarin metabolism?	Induces warfarin metabolism, thereby decreasing warfarin blood levels
What happens to the INR of warfarin patients who begin thyroid replacement medication?	INR increases; thyroid hormone increases the metabolism of clotting factors, thereby potentiating the effects of warfarin
What happens to the INR of warfarin patients who begin antimicrobial therapy with sulfonamides?	INR increases; sulfonamides inhibit CYP-450 2C9, thereby increasing warfarin levels
Does warfarin cross the placental barrier?	Yes (contraindicated in pregnancy); warfarin is teratogenic
What are the adverse effects of warfarin?	Bleeding; drug-drug interactions; skin necrosis (seen within the first few days of warfarin therapy and is secondary to decreased protein C levels); "purple toes syndrome" (caused by cholesterol microembolization)
What can be used to counteract the effects of warfarin?	Vitamin K (slow onset); fresh frozen plasma (rapid onset)

How is warfarin metabolized?   Hepatic cytochrome P-450 enzymes

The synthesis of what two factors is inhibited first when warfarin therapy is initiated?
1. Factor VII
2. Protein C (therefore patients may initially be hypercoagulable when warfarin is first initiated)

Why are factor VII and protein C inhibited first when warfarin therapy is initiated?   These proteins have the shortest half-lives when compared to the half-lives of factors II, IX, X, and protein S

What is the mechanism of action of abciximab, eptifibatide, and tirofiban?   Blockade of the glycoprotein IIb/IIIa receptor on platelets, thereby inhibiting platelet aggregation

What is the physiologic ligand for the glycoprotein IIb/IIIa receptor?   Fibrinogen

What is the mechanism of action of thrombolytic agents?   Conversion of plasminogen to plasmin; plasmin cleaves fibrin, thereby leading to lysis of thrombi

What is the main adverse effect of thrombolytic agents?   Hemorrhage

Thrombolytic agents are contraindicated in what settings?   Active internal bleeding; history of cerebrovascular accident (CVA); recent intracranial or intraspinal surgery; intracranial neoplasm; AV malformation; severe uncontrolled HTN (systolic blood pressure [SBP] >185 mm Hg or diastolic blood pressure [DBP] >110 mm Hg); evidence of intracranial hemorrhage; suspected aortic dissection; seizure at the onset of stroke; current use of anticoagulants or an INR >1.7; lumbar puncture within 1 week

What are the therapeutic indications of thrombolytic therapy?   Acute MI; acute PE; acute ischemic stroke

What is the "therapeutic time window" for administering thrombolytic agents to patients with acute ischemic stroke?   Within the first 3 hours of the onset of symptoms

Give examples of thrombolytic agents: Alteplase; anistreplase; streptokinase; urokinase

What two drugs can counteract thrombolytic agent therapy?
1. Aminocaproic acid
2. Tranexamic acid (both agents inhibit plasminogen activation)

With regard to thrombolytic agents, what does "clot-specific" mean?	The drug specifically activates plasminogen that is bound to fibrin in a thrombus with a low affinity for free, circulating plasminogen
Which thrombolytic agent is "clot-specific"?	Alteplase
Alteplase is also known as what?	tPA (tissue plasminogen activator)
What is the half-life of tPA?	5 minutes
Where does tPA come from?	Recombinant DNA technology
What type of enzymatic activity does tPA possess?	Serine protease activity
Where does streptokinase come from?	Group C β-hemolytic streptococci
How does streptokinase work as a thrombolytic agent?	Forms a 1:1 complex with plasminogen; complexed plasminogen then converts free plasminogen into plasmin (active form)
Does streptokinase have any enzymatic activity?	No
Is streptokinase "clot-specific"?	No
What other proteins does the streptokinase-plasminogen complex degrade?	Fibrinogen; factor V; factor VII
What laboratory value is monitored with streptokinase therapy?	Thromboplastin time
Why is streptokinase antigenic?	It is recognized as a foreign protein (antigen).
What adverse reactions are specific to streptokinase?	Anaphylaxis; rash; fever
What is the half-life of anistreplase?	90 minutes
How does anistreplase work as a thrombolytic?	Anisoyl group blocks the active site of plasminogen; as complex binds to fibrin, anisoyl group is removed and the complex becomes activated.
Does urokinase have enzymatic activity?	Yes

Originally, where did urokinase come from?	Human urine
Where does urokinase come from now?	Fetal renal cells (human)
Is urokinase antigenic?	No, since it is not a foreign protein.
Will streptokinase, at normal doses, work in patients with a recent history of streptococcal infection?	No, because antibodies made against recent streptococcal antigens will bind to and inactivate streptokinase.

CLINICAL VIGNETTES

A 72-year-old man with a past medical history of CHF presents to the emergency room with colicky right-sided flank pain. Renal ultrasonography shows a 5 mm calculus in the right ureter. What medication is the patient likely on that has exacerbated this situation? What medication could the patient be switched to?

Furosemide and other loop diuretics are frequently employed in the treatment of CHF to help decrease preload to the heart and vascular congestion that can cause pulmonary edema. However, loop diuretics increase the urinary excretion of calcium which can lead to renal stone formation. As this patient is presenting with a stone, if his CHF symptoms can be controlled on an alternative agent, the loop diuretics should be discontinued. A thiazide diuretic, such as hydrochlorothiazide, may provide adequate diuresis to control his CHF symptoms, while at the same time decreasing urinary calcium excretion, preventing further stone formation.

A 32-year-old woman is found to have a deep venous thrombosis (DVT) in her right calf and therapy is started with heparin bridging therapy with close monitoring of her activated partial thromboplastin time. Warfarin is added to the therapy, with the goal of discontinuing heparin once the patient reaches a therapeutic INR. A repeat Doppler ultrasonography of the right calf after 1 week of therapy unexpectedly shows expansion of the clot. What is likely to be found on this patient's complete blood count (CBC), and what is the appropriate therapy?

Paradoxical clot expansion or new clot formation is most likely the result of heparin-induced thrombocytopenia (HIT) in this patient. HIT is a rare complication seen after at least 7 days of treatment with unfractionated heparin. Heparin molecules induce the formation of antiheparin antibodies (IgG). These antibodies bind to heparin and platelet factor 4, causing platelet activation and aggregation, with a subsequent drop in platelet numbers. Therefore, the CBC will reveal a low platelet count. Heparin therapy should be stopped immediately. Low-molecular-weight heparins such as enoxaparin are contraindicated in patients with a history of HIT, and therefore would not be appropriate alternative therapy in this patient. Here, we could measure the patient's INR, and if therapeutic, warfarin monotherapy could be continued for 3 to 6 months. Alternative anticoagulation therapies available to patients with HIT include lepirudin, a factor IIa inhibitor, and argatroban, a synthetic direct thrombin inhibitor.

A 63-year-old man who is being treated for hypercholesterolemia with an HMG-CoA reductase inhibitor (a statin) comes in for a follow-up visit. He began taking the medication 1 week ago. He is complaining of some mild muscle aches and pains, which he attributes to the new exercise regimen he just started on your recommendation. Laboratory studies show a minor increase in creatine kinase (CK) activity. He asks if the new medication could be causing this pain, and if he should stop taking the medication. How should the physician advise the patient?

Statin myopathy is a concerning but relatively rare complication of statin therapy, with an incident of 0.1% to 0.5%. Rhabdomyolysis due to statin therapy is notably less common. Rhabdomyolysis is an indication for immediate cessation of statin therapy, but myopathy is not necessarily. Myopathy usually manifests within 1 week of starting a statin, and is dose dependent. If statin therapy is successful in lowering serum cholesterol, and CK elevation is not significantly elevated above baseline, lowering the dose of the medication or switching to a different statin may be appropriate. A controversial topic is the use of coenzyme Q10 (CoQ10), or ubiquinone, to treat and prevent statin-induced myopathy. Statins also inhibit the reaction that forms CoQ10. CoQ10 is found in the mitochondria of many cell types and is an antioxidant that might maintain muscle health. It has been shown in limited studies to decrease muscle pain in patients taking statins. Its long-term safety and efficacy are yet unknown.

CHAPTER 7

Pulmonary Agents

DRUGS FOR ASTHMA

What are the classifications of asthma severity?	Mild intermittent; mild persistent; moderate persistent; severe persistent
What are the main classifications of drugs for asthma?	Bronchodilators; anti-inflammatory agents

Name the drug class for each of the following medications:

Albuterol	Short-acting β_2-adrenergic agonist
Epinephrine	Short-acting β_2-adrenergic agonist
Terbutaline	Short-acting β_2-adrenergic agonist
Salmeterol	Long-acting β_2-adrenergic agonist
Formoterol	Long-acting β_2-adrenergic agonist
Isoproterenol	Short-acting β-adrenergic agonist
Metaproterenol	Short-acting β-adrenergic agonist
Fluticasone	Inhaled corticosteroid
Flunisolide	Inhaled corticosteroid
Beclomethasone	Inhaled corticosteroid
Triamcinolone	Inhaled corticosteroid
Budesonide	Inhaled corticosteroid
Methylprednisolone	Systemic corticosteroid
Prednisone	Systemic corticosteroid
Cromolyn	Mast cell stabilizer
Nedocromil	Mast cell stabilizer
Ipratropium	Inhaled anticholinergic
Tiotropium	Inhaled anticholinergic
Theophylline	Phosphodiesterase inhibitor; adenosine antagonist; methylxanthine
Zileuton	5-Lipoxygenase inhibitor
Zafirlukast	Leukotriene receptor antagonist
Montelukast	Leukotriene receptor antagonist

How do β_2-agonists help treat asthma?

Bronchodilation via β_2-adrenoceptor-mediated smooth muscle relaxation

How do corticosteroids help treat asthma?

Decrease production and release of proinflammatory cytokines; decrease inflammatory cell activation, recruitment, and infiltration; decrease vascular permeability; decrease mucous production; increase number and sensitivity of β_2-adrenergic receptors

How do mast cell stabilizers help treat asthma?

Prevent mast cell degranulation, thereby decreasing release of histamine, platelet activating factor, leukotrienes, and other mediators that cause bronchoconstriction. Therefore only useful before exposure to allergen.

How do inhaled anticholinergics help treat asthma?

Competitively inhibit muscarinic receptors, thereby inhibiting vagal-mediated bronchoconstriction; reduce mucous production

How do phosphodiesterase inhibitors help treat asthma?

Increase cAMP which causes bronchodilation

How do 5-lipoxygenase inhibitors help treat asthma?

Inhibits production of leukotrienes (LTC_4, LTD_4, LTE_4) from arachidonic acid, thereby preventing bronchoconstriction

What β_2-adrenergic agonist is commonly used as a tocolytic agent (stops premature labor by relaxing uterine smooth muscle)?

Terbutaline

What cation can be used as a tocolytic agent?

Mg^{2+} (Magnesium ion)

Is cromolyn used for treatment or prevention of an asthma attack?

Prevention

Is nedocromil effective during an acute asthma attack?

No

What are the side effects of mast cell stabilizers?

Bitter taste; throat irritation

What are the side effects of β_2-adrenergic agonists?	Tachycardia; muscle tremors; anxiety; arrhythmias; hyperglycemia; hypokalemia; hypomagnesemia (systemic side effects are minimized when drug is delivered via inhalation)
What are the side effects of 5-lipoxygenase inhibitors and leukotriene antagonists?	Increased liver function tests (LFTs); headache; Churg-Strauss syndrome
What is the main nonsystemic side effect of inhaled corticosteroids?	Thrush
What is thrush?	Oropharyngeal candidiasis
How can you prevent thrush when using inhaled corticosteroids?	Use of a spacer device; rinse mouth with water after medication use
What is a possible systemic side effect of inhaled corticosteroids in children?	Decreased growth of long bones
If using an inhaled corticosteroid and β_2-adrenergic agonist together, which do you use first?	β_2-adrenergic agonist (bronchodilates the airways, thereby increasing amount of corticosteroid that is delivered to its site of action)
What are the side effects of theophylline?	Tachycardia; arrhythmias; nausea; diarrhea; central nervous system (CNS) excitation (narrow therapeutic index)
Give an example of a methylxanthine other than theophylline:	Caffeine; theobromine; aminophylline
Why do inhaled anticholinergics have a minimal side effect profile?	Quaternary ammonium derivatives of atropine, therefore, do not leave the pulmonary system and cannot cross the blood-brain barrier
What are examples of systemic anticholinergic side effects?	Dry mouth; dry eyes; constipation; urinary retention; blurred vision; mydriasis; drowsiness; tachycardia
How do you treat β-blocker-induced bronchospasm?	With anticholinergics such as ipratropium and tiotropium
Name two drugs used to treat an acute asthma attack:	1. Epinephrine 2. Albuterol
What is the IV form of theophylline called?	Aminophylline (2:1 complex of theophylline and ethylenediamine)

What is the term used to describe a severe asthma attack that does not respond to usual asthma therapy?	Status asthmaticus
How is status asthmaticus treated?	Oxygen; inhaled albuterol; intravenous or oral corticosteroids; inhaled anticholinergics
What is the drug of choice for mild asthma?	Short-acting β_2-adrenergic agonist
What is the maintenance drug of choice for chronic asthma?	Inhaled glucocorticoid
How is theophylline primarily metabolized?	Hepatic cytochrome P-450 enzymes (CYP 1A2 and CYP 3A4)
Give examples of medications that can lead to increased theophylline levels when used concomitantly:	Cimetidine; erythromycin; fluoroquinolones
What drug can cause asthma, nasal polyps, and rhinitis?	Aspirin ("aspirin triad"); seen in the rare case of aspirin sensitivity where inhibition of cyclooxygenase (COX) leads to a buildup of leukotrienes

CHRONIC OBSTRUCTIVE PULMONARY DISEASE AGENTS

What disease processes fall under the category of chronic obstructive pulmonary disease (COPD)?	Asthma; chronic bronchitis; emphysema
State whether the following pulmonary function tests (PFTs) will be increased, decreased, or remain unchanged in patients with COPD:	
Forced expiratory volume in 1 second (FEV$_1$)	Decreased
Forced vital capacity (FVC)	Unchanged or increased
FEV$_1$/FVC	Decreased (<75%)
Total lung capacity (TLC)	Unchanged or increased
What agents are used to treat COPD?	Inhaled anticholinergics; β_2-adrenergic agonists; theophylline; inhaled corticosteroids
What are the first-line agents for treatment of COPD?	Inhaled anticholinergics (ipratropium)

ANTITUSSIVE AGENTS

Give examples of drugs that can suppress the CNS cough reflex:	Morphine; codeine; hydrocodone; hydromorphone; dextromethorphan
Which has greater antitussive (anticough) action, morphine or codeine?	Codeine
When using opioids for cough suppression, are the doses required less than, equal to, or greater than the doses required for analgesic activity?	Less than
Which opioid is the drug of choice for cough suppression?	Dextromethorphan (no analgesic activity, no addiction risk)
What is a cough expectorant?	An agent that thins respiratory tract mucus and promotes its expulsion from the tracheobronchial system
Give an example of a cough expectorant:	Guaifenesin

AGENTS FOR ALLERGIC RHINITIS

What is/are the signs and symptoms of allergic rhinitis?	Inflammation of the nasal mucous membrane which is characterized by nasal itching, sneezing, rhinorrhea, and congestion
What causes allergic rhinitis?	Allergens interacting with IgE-coated mast cells leading to release of histamine, leukotrienes, and chemotactic factors
How do you treat allergic rhinitis?	Antihistamines; α-adrenergic agonists; intranasal corticosteroids; intranasal cromolyn; 5-lipoxygenase inhibitors; leukotriene antagonists
Give examples of antihistamines used in the treatment of allergic rhinitis:	Diphenhydramine; chlorpheniramine; loratadine; desloratadine; fexofenadine; cetirizine; astemizole

Name three nonsedating antihistamines:	1. Loratadine 2. Desloratadine 3. Fexofenadine
Why are loratadine, desloratadine, and fexofenadine nonsedating?	No CNS entry
Where are H_1 histamine receptors located?	Smooth muscle; endothelial cells; heart; CNS

Histamine acting at H_1 receptors does what to the following?

Bronchiolar smooth muscle	Contraction
Capillaries	Dilation; increased permeability
Peripheral nociceptive receptors	Activation which leads to increased pruritus and pain
What are the major side effects of diphenhydramine?	Anticholinergic side effects, such as sedation, dry mouth, dry eyes, constipation, urinary retention, blurred vision, mydriasis, and tachycardia
Give examples of α-adrenergic agonists (nasal decongestants) used in the treatment of allergic rhinitis:	Phenylephrine; pseudoephedrine; oxymetazoline
How do α-adrenergic agonists help relieve signs and symptoms of allergic rhinitis?	Vasoconstriction of dilated arterioles in nasal mucosa; decrease airway resistance
What can happen when you discontinue use of long-term intranasal decongestants?	Rebound nasal congestion (only use these types of medications for short-term relief)

AGENTS FOR RESPIRATORY DISTRESS SYNDROME

What causes neonatal respiratory distress syndrome?	Insufficient maturation of type II pneumocytes leading to decreased production of surfactant
What is the purpose of lung surfactant?	Reduce alveolar surface tension which allows alveoli to remain open for proper gas exchange
What medications can be used to accelerate fetal lung maturation?	Glucocorticoids; thyrotropin-releasing-hormone (TRH)

What is a marker of fetal lung maturity?

Lecithin to sphingomyelin ratio of at least 1.5:1

What pharmacologic options are available for treating neonatal respiratory distress syndrome?

Surfactant replacement therapy; nitric oxide (NO)

AGENTS FOR CYSTIC FIBROSIS

What can be used to reduce small airway accumulation of viscous mucus in cystic fibrosis patients?

N-acetylcysteine; DNase

How does *N*-acetylcysteine work in cystic fibrosis?

Acts as a mucolytic agent through its free sulfhydryl group which breaks disulfide bonds in mucoproteins, thereby lowering mucus viscosity

How does DNase work in cystic fibrosis?

Deoxyribonuclease that selectively cleaves polymerized DNA in pulmonary secretions, thereby reducing mucus viscosity

Patients receiving which radiologic enhancing compound can be given concomitant *N*-acetylcysteine to protect renal function?

Computed tomography (CT) contrast

CLINICAL VIGNETTES

A 62-year-old man with a 40 pack-year smoking history presents to your office complaining of progressive shortness of breath. He has been using his niece's albuterol inhaler with minimal relief of his symptoms. Visual inspection of the patient shows an increased anterior-posterior diameter of the chest. Auscultation of the lungs reveals a prolonged expiratory phase and pulmonary function tests reveal a decreased FEV_1/FVC ratio. The patient shows mildly increased work of breathing after walking to the examination room, and exhales through pursed lips. Why has the albuterol therapy failed to relieve his shortness of breath?

This patient is suffering from COPD, a diagnosis supported by his long smoking history and physical findings. He appears to have a large emphysemic component to his disease. Emphysema is a pathologic diagnosis characterized by the destruction of alveolar tissue. Because of the destruction of the pulmonary parenchyma, oxygen exchange, and not oxygen delivery is the main issue for the patient. Therefore, a bronchodilator such as albuterol is minimally effective. COPD is characteristically an obstructive respiratory process that is nonresponsive to bronchodilators. This is in contrast to asthma, an obstructive pulmonary disease that is bronchodilator responsive.

A 12-year-old girl with a past medical history of asthma and allergic rhinitis presents with worsening asthma symptoms. She is now using her rescue inhaler every day for asthma exacerbations. She also awakens two to three times per week at night with shortness of breath and chest tightness. In the office, her peak flow volume measures 80% of the volume on her previous visit, when she had been feeling well. What is the most appropriate recommendation at this time?

This patient meets the criteria for moderate persistent asthma. Her symptoms are no longer being controlled on her albuterol rescue inhaler alone. Her history of allergic rhinitis suggests an allergic component to her asthma, so fastidious allergen avoidance is necessary. However, it is also appropriate at this time to add additional pharmacologic therapy to control her symptoms. An inhaled corticosteroid should be added to reduce airway inflammation and to prevent airway remodeling. Inhaled corticosteroids do not treat acute exacerbations, but decrease the frequency of attacks when taken regularly. The addition of a long-acting β_2-adrenergic agonist such as salmeterol or formoterol could also be considered.

A mother brings in her 8-year-old boy who has been suffering from minor cold symptoms for 1 day with a cough that kept the child from sleeping well last night. After assuring the mother that the child has a minor viral illness that will not respond to antibiotics, you suggest over-the-counter Robitussin to control the coughing. The mother asks you about the active ingredient in the medication. You respond that the active ingredient is dextromethorphan, an opioid medication that is effective for cough suppression. The mother becomes quite agitated that you would suggest an addictive substance for her young child. What is the most appropriate counseling in this situation?

Dextromethorphan is the most widely used antitussive agent and has been available in various over-the-counter (OTC) preparations since the 1950s. It has the advantage over codeine of having less addictive potential and causing less constipation. It is FDA approved for OTC cough and cold formulations for children over the age of 6. Therefore, the mother can be counseled that this is a very safe medication with little to no addictive potential and will be effective in relieving her child's symptoms. However, she must feel comfortable with her child's therapy, and if this information does not assuage her fears, alternative therapies should be discussed. It is also true that while physiologic dependence does not occur in this agent to the level of other narcotic drugs, cough medications containing dextromethorphan are nevertheless used as a drug of abuse, especially in adolescent populations.

CHAPTER 8

Gastrointestinal Agents

AGENTS FOR GASTROESOPHAGEAL REFLUX DISEASE

What is the main cause of gastroesophageal reflux disease (GERD)?

Decreased lower esophageal sphincter pressure

What complications may arise from GERD?

Strictures; esophagitis; Barrett esophagus (squamocolumnar metaplasia)

What are the drug therapy goals in treating GERD?

To eliminate symptoms; heal esophagitis; prevent the relapse of esophagitis; prevent the development of complications

What types of medications may be useful in the treatment of GERD?

Antacids; H_2-receptor antagonists; proton pump inhibitors (PPIs); prokinetic agents (cisapride, metoclopramide, bethanechol); mucosal protectants (sucralfate)

Give the mechanism of action for each of the following drugs or drug classes:

Antacids	Weak bases that increase gastric pH through acid-neutralizing ability to form a salt and water
H_2-receptor antagonists	Competitively antagonize H_2 receptors on gastric parietal cells, thereby decreasing acid production
PPIs	Inhibit gastric acid secretion via inhibiting gastric parietal cell H^+/K^+-ATPase. Restoration of acid secretion requires resynthesis of the H^+/K^+-ATPase (proton pump).
• Cisapride	• Increases lower esophageal sphincter pressure; accelerate gastric emptying time; increases amplitude of esophageal contractions; 5-HT_4 agonist; 5-HT_3 antagonist
Metoclopramide	Dopamine (D_2) receptor antagonist; increases lower esophageal sphincter pressure; accelerates gastric emptying time
Sucralfate	When exposed to acid, complexes with positively charged proteins to form a viscous coat, thereby protecting gastric lining from gastric acid secretions

What are the adverse effects caused by metoclopramide?	Anxiety; insomnia; extrapyramidal symptoms; increased prolactin levels
What are the adverse effects caused by sucralfate?	Constipation; nausea; abdominal discomfort
What are the possible adverse effects of antacids?	Belching (sodium bicarbonate and calcium carbonate); diarrhea (magnesium salts); constipation (calcium or aluminum salts); acid-base disturbances; bone damage via binding phosphate in the gut (aluminum salts); worsening of hypertension and congestive heart failure (CHF) (sodium salts); decreased absorption of medications via pH alteration or formation of insoluble complexes (tetracycline, fluoroquinolones, isoniazid [INH], ferrous sulfate, ketoconazole, PPIs)

Which antacid(s) can produce a metabolic alkalosis?	Sodium bicarbonate; calcium carbonate
What causes the milk-alkali syndrome?	Ingestion of excessive amounts of calcium and absorbable alkali such as sodium bicarbonate or calcium carbonate
What is a potential complication after discontinuing chronic antacid use?	Acid rebound
List the names of the H_2-receptor antagonists:	Cimetidine; famotidine; ranitidine; nizatidine
Which H_2-receptor antagonist inhibits hepatic cytochrome P-450 metabolizing enzymes?	Cimetidine
Name at least five drugs showing potential drug interactions with cimetidine:	1. Warfarin 2. Diazepam 3. Phenytoin 4. Metronidazole 5. Propranolol 6. Lidocaine 7. Calcium channel blockers (CCBs) 8. Theophylline 9. Certain tricyclic antidepressants (TCAs); chlordiazepoxide
Which H_2-receptor antagonist can cause gynecomastia?	Cimetidine (prolactin-stimulating activity)
Which H_2-receptor antagonist has antiandrogenic activity?	Cimetidine
List the names of the PPIs:	Omeprazole; esomeprazole; lansoprazole; rabeprazole; pantoprazole
What are the common side effects of PPIs?	Headache; dizziness; nausea; diarrhea; constipation. Prolonged use can lead to bacterial overgrowth in the GI tract. Note also that a recent analysis revealed that people (age $\geq$ 50) taking high doses of PPIs for more than a year were 2.6 times as likely to break a hip as were people not taking PPIs. Histamine H_2-receptor inhibitors also increased fracture risk, but not to the extent as did PPIs.

What is the most serious side effect of cisapride?

Prolongation of the QT interval

Cisapride should be avoided in which type of patients?

Patients with prolonged QT intervals; patients taking medications that inhibit cytochrome P-450 3A4 (fluconazole, ketoconazole, itraconazole, erythromycin, clarithromycin, ritonavir)

What arrhythmia can be caused by prolongation of the QT interval?

Torsades de pointes (a polymorphic ventricular tachycardia)

Which drugs increase cisapride blood levels by inhibiting the cytochrome P-450 3A4 enzymes that metabolize cisapride? (Please mention at least four drugs).

1. Erythromycin
2. Clarithromycin
3. Itraconazole
4. Fluconazole
5. Ketoconazole
6. Indinavir
7. Ritonavir
8. Class 1A antiarrhythmics
9. Class III antiarrhythmics
10. Certain TCAs
11. Certain antipsychotics

AGENTS FOR PEPTIC ULCER DISEASE

What three mediators can stimulate acid secretion from parietal cells?

1. Acetylcholine
2. Histamine (via H_2 receptor)
3. Gastrin

Name three causes of peptic ulcer disease (PUD):

1. *Helicobacter pylori* infection (primary cause)
2. Nonsteroidal anti-inflammatory drugs (NSAIDs)
3. Extreme physiologic stress (ie, patients in the ICU setting being ventilated, burn patients)

What type of patients do acute peptic ulcers occur in?

Hospitalized patients who are critically ill (stress ulcers)

What is the name of the syndrome that is characterized by hypersecretion of gastric acid secondary to a gastrin-secreting tumor?

Zollinger-Ellison syndrome

Which are the drug therapy goals in treating PUD?

Control *H. pylori* infection; alleviate symptoms; promote healing; prevent recurrences; prevent complications (eg, hemorrhage)

What types of medications are useful for the treatment of PUD?

Antimicrobial agents; H$_2$-receptor antagonists; PPIs; prostaglandins; antimuscarinic agents; antacids; mucosal protective agents; bismuth salts

How might *H. pylori* play a role in peptic ulcer development?

Direct mucosal damage; alterations in inflammatory response; induced hypergastrinemia

Meals worsen the pain associated with what type of ulcer?

Gastric ulcer

Meals relieve the pain associated with what type of ulcer?

Duodenal ulcer

What treatment options are available to eradicate *H. pylori*?

Triple therapy with a PPI added to two antimicrobial agents such as metronidazole, amoxicillin, tetracycline, or clarithromycin; four-drug regimens consisting of triple therapy plus bismuth subsalicylate; (must use triple or quadruple antibiotic therapy to eradicate *H. pylori*)

Why should you not give bismuth subsalicylate to children?

- May be associated with Reye syndrome (contains salicylates)

What is Reye syndrome?

Acute onset encephalopathy and fatty liver formation. Symptoms begin with vomiting, lethargy, and confusion progressing to stupor, respiratory distress, coma, and seizures. Its cause is unknown, but has been found to be associated with aspirin use in young children. Therefore, aspirin administration is to be avoided in pediatric patients.

How do prostaglandins help treat PUD?

Prostaglandins such as PGE$_2$ and PGI$_2$ inhibit gastric acid secretion and stimulate secretion of bicarbonate and mucus (cytoprotective activity); used to treat NSAID-induced peptic ulcers

Which prostaglandin analog is commonly used as a cytoprotective agent for the treatment of PUD?

Misoprostol (synthetic PGE$_1$ analog)

Why should misoprostol not be given to a preterm pregnant woman?

Induction of premature uterine contractions (abortifacient properties)

AGENTS FOR INFLAMMATORY BOWEL DISEASE

What are the two forms of inflammatory bowel disease (IBD)?

1. Crohn disease
2. Ulcerative colitis (UC)

Does treatment of IBD cure or control the disease process?

Control

What types of medications are used to treat IBD?

Corticosteroids; aminosalicylates; immunosuppressives; monoclonal antibodies

Sulfasalazine is cleaved by gut bacteria in the colon to produce what two compounds?

1. Sulfapyridine (sulfonamide antibiotic)
2. Mesalamine (5-aminosalicylic acid, 5-ASA)

What is the active component of sulfasalazine for IBD?

Mesalamine or 5-ASA; 5-ASA is the metabolite active against IBD, while sulfapyridine is the metabolite active against rheumatoid arthritis. Formulation into sulfasalazine is necessary to prevent rapid proximal gut absorption so that sufficient 5-ASA is delivered to the distal gut to effectively treat IBD.

How does mesalamine work in the treatment of IBD?

Anti-inflammatory effects; immunomodulating effects

What type of vitamin supplementation should patients receive while on sulfasalazine?

Folic acid since sulfasalazine may interfere with absorption of folic acid in the gut, leading to megaloblastic anemia

What types of immunosuppressives are used to treat IBD?

Cyclosporine A; methotrexate; azathioprine; 6-mercaptopurine

What is the name of the monoclonal antibody indicated for the treatment of Crohn disease?

Infliximab

What is infliximab's mechanism of action?

Monoclonal antibody that binds to soluble and bound forms of tumor necrosis factor-alpha (TNF-α)

True or False? Once remission has been achieved with ulcerative colitis, corticosteroids are used as maintenance therapy.

False. Corticosteroids should not be used to maintain disease remission due to their high systemic toxicity. Aminosalicylates or immunosuppressive agents are used for maintenance therapy for UC.

AGENTS FOR NAUSEA AND VOMITING

Name a major chemosensory area for emesis:	Chemoreceptor trigger zone (CTZ)
Where is the CTZ found?	Area postrema of the fourth ventricle of the brain
Give examples of drug classes that are effective in the treatment of nausea and vomiting:	Antihistamine-anticholinergics; benzodiazepines; butyrophenones; cannabinoids; corticosteroids; phenothiazines; substituted benzamides; 5-HT$_3$-receptor antagonists; neurokinin receptor antagonists

Give examples of specific drugs in each of the following drug classes used in the treatment of nausea and vomiting:

Antihistamine-anticholinergics	Diphenhydramine; hydroxyzine; meclizine; cyclizine; promethazine; pyrilamine; scopolamine; trimethobenzamide
Benzodiazepines	Alprazolam; diazepam; lorazepam
Butyrophenones	Haloperidol; droperidol; domperidone
Cannabinoids	Dronabinol; nabilone
Corticosteroids	Dexamethasone; methylprednisolone
Phenothiazines	Prochlorperazine; chlorpromazine; perphenazine
Substituted benzamides	Metoclopramide
5-HT$_3$-receptor antagonists	Ondansetron; dolasetron; granisetron
Neurokinin receptor antagonists	Aprepitant (oral); fosaprepitant (IV formulation converted to aprepitant)

Do synthetic cannabinoids have psychotropic activity?	No
How does metoclopramide work as an antiemetic?	Blocks dopamine receptors centrally in the CTZ
What is intractable emesis leading to dehydration and hypotension during pregnancy called?	Hyperemesis gravidarum

What are the drugs of choice for treating emesis during pregnancy?	Meclizine; cyclizine; promethazine
What antihistamine is often used to treat motion sickness?	Meclizine
What anticholinergic is often used to treat motion sickness?	Scopolamine
How is scopolamine normally administered?	As a transdermal patch to prevent systemic anticholinergic effects
What medication is often used in combination regimens to enhance antiemetic activity?	Dexamethasone
What are the side effects of cannabinoids?	Anxiety; memory loss; confusion; motor incoordination; hallucinations; euphoria; relaxation; hunger; gynecomastia
What are the side effects of the phenothiazine antiemetics?	Extrapyramidal symptoms; sedation; hypotension
Why doesn't ondansetron cause extrapyramidal side effects?	Blocks 5-HT$_3$ instead of dopamine receptors in the CTZ
What chemotherapy agent has one of the highest emetogenic potentials?	Cisplatin
What over-the-counter (OTC) medication can be given in combination with metoclopramide to reduce its extrapyramidal side effects?	Diphenhydramine can be used for its anticholinergic properties. EPS symptoms with metoclopramide use are due to central dopamine receptor blockade, and tardive dyskinesia, if it develops, may be irreversible. Therefore, metoclopramide should only be used for short-term therapy if possible.
What macrolide antibiotic also has prokinetic properties for the GI tract?	Erythromycin, though tolerance to this effect develops rapidly, limiting its usefulness

AGENTS FOR DIARRHEA AND CONSTIPATION

Name three classes of drugs that are effective in the treatment of diarrhea:	1. Adsorbents 2. Antimotility agents 3. Antisecretory agents

Define adsorbent:

A substance offering a suitable active surface, upon which other substances may adhere to

Give examples of specific drugs in each of the following drug classes used in the treatment of diarrhea:

    Adsorbents

Kaolin; pectin; polycarbophil; attapulgite

    Antimotility agents

Diphenoxylate; loperamide; morphine

    Antisecretory agents

Bismuth subsalicylate

Give the antidiarrheal mechanism of action for each of the following drug classes:

    Adsorbents

Adsorbs (adheres to) drugs, nutrients, toxins, and digestive juices

    Antimotility agents

Decrease peristalsis by activating presynaptic opioid receptors in the enteric nervous system

    Antisecretory agents

Decrease fluid secretion in the bowel

What adsorbent can absorb 60 times its weight in water and treat both diarrhea and constipation?

Polycarbophil

What are the potential side effects of bismuth subsalicylate?

Salicylism (tinnitus, nausea, vomiting); darkening of tongue; darkening of stools; induce gout attacks in susceptible patients

What antidiarrheal can decrease tetracycline absorption if given concomitantly?

Bismuth subsalicylate

What antidiarrheal is often formulated in combination with atropine?

Diphenoxylate

Which class of antidiarrheals can cause paralytic ileus?

Antimotility agents

What medication is often used to treat flushing and diarrhea seen in carcinoid syndrome and vasoactive intestinal peptide secreting tumors (VIPomas)?

Octreotide

What is octreotide's mechanism of action?	Synthetic analog of somatostatin which blocks release of serotonin and other vasoactive peptides; direct inhibitory effects on intestinal secretion; direct stimulatory effects on intestinal absorption
What are the non-antidiarrheal uses of octreotide?	Esophageal varices; acromegaly
What medication can be used in conjunction with antibiotics to bulk stools and absorb *Clostridium difficile* toxins A and B in *C. difficile* colitis?	Cholestyramine, a nonabsorbable binding agent
What types of medications cause constipation?	Opioid analgesics; anticholinergics; calcium-containing antacids; aluminum-containing antacids; calcium channel blockers; clonidine; iron; sodium polystyrene sulfonate
Give examples of drug classes that are effective in the treatment of constipation:	Bulk forming agents; irritants and stimulants; stool softeners
Give examples of specific drugs in each of the following drug classes used in the treatment of constipation:	
Bulk forming agents	Methylcellulose; psyllium; bran; magnesium-containing salts; polyethylene glycol
Osmotic laxatives	Lactulose; magnesium hydroxide (milk of magnesia); sorbitol; magnesium citrate; sodium phosphate; polyethylene glycol
Irritants and stimulants	Cascara; senna; aloe; bisacodyl
Stool softeners	Mineral oil; docusate (oral or enema, trade name: Colace); glycerin suppository
Cl⁻ channel activators	Lubiprostone (Amitiza)

Give the mechanism of action for each
of the following drug classes:

Bulk-forming agents	Form gels in large intestine which causes water retention and intestinal distention, thereby increasing peristaltic activity
Osmotic laxatives	Nonabsorbable compounds which draw fluid into the colon to maintain osmotic neutrality
Irritants and stimulants	Irritate gut lining which subsequently increases peristalsis
Stool softeners	Surfactants that become emulsified with stool, thereby softening feces
Cl⁻ channel activators	Activate CIC-2 Cl⁻ channels in the apical membrane of intestinal cells increasing fluid and intestinal motility without altering serum Na^+ or K^+ levels. The effects are localized to the GI tract, increase fluid secretion into the intestinal lumen, and accelerate fecal transit.
What are the potential side effects of bisacodyl?	Abdominal cramping; atonic colon

CLINICAL VIGNETTES

A 50-year-old woman is in the surgical intensive care unit (ICU) status post right middle cerebral artery hemorrhagic stroke. She is being mechanically ventilated. Her morning laboratories come back with a platelet count of 50,000 (normal 150,000-450,000). Given her history, she is not on deep venous thrombosis (DVT) prophylaxis with heparin. What other prophylactic medication, commonly employed in a critical care setting, may be responsible for her drop in platelet count?

Patients in ICUs are routinely put on DVT and GI prophylaxis given the prolonged immobility and high physiologic stress of intensive care. Pharmacologic DVT prophylaxis is not appropriate in this patient, and mechanical methods such as sequential compression stockings should be used instead. However, this patient was most likely started on omeprazole for prevention of stress-induced gastric ulcers. Omeprazole can cause thrombocytopenia. This patient should be switched to a different GI prophylactic medication. Esomeprazole, the S-enantiomer of omeprazole, while controversial as to whether or not it is more effective to inhibit stomach acid secretion, does not carry the same risk of lowering platelets.

A 60-year-old woman with a past medical history of rheumatoid arthritis (RA) and chronic iron deficiency anemia is found to have blood in her stool. Colonoscopy is negative, but a gastric ulceration is discovered upon upper endoscopy. After successful treatment of the ulcer, what medication could be added to the patient's regimen to prevent a repeat ulcer or gastric perforation?

Patients with a chronic inflammatory disease such as RA are often successful in relieving their pain symptoms with long-term treatment with NSAIDs. However, this therapy can lead to gastric ulceration and chronic gastrointestinal bleeding that can lead to iron deficiency anemia. This anemia is often overlooked in patients with chronic autoimmune disorders as anemia of chronic disease. All GI bleeding must be considered colon cancer until proven otherwise, especially in patients older than 50 years, but once ruled out the next most likely location in this patient is a gastric ulcer due to disruption of the gastric mucosa by long-term NSAID administration. Because of the patient's RA, NSAID cessation is difficult. In patients such as this, addition of misoprostol, a prostaglandin analog, may be appropriate.

An 86-year-old woman with a history of chronic constipation is treated with lactulose with good relief of her constipation. However, she complains of painful abdominal cramps and embarrassing flatus and wishes to try another medication. What laxative has a similar mechanism of action to lactulose and will not cause large electrolyte imbalances, making it safe to use in this elderly patient?

Polyethylene glycol (PEG) is an osmotic laxative used in high concentration formulas as a bowel cleanser prior to endoscopic procedures. It is effective in lower concentrations for treatment of chronic constipation. Unlike lactulose and sorbitol, it is not metabolized by colonic bacteria, decreasing colonic gas formation. It does not cause large fluid or electrolyte shifts. Therefore, unlike magnesium citrate, sodium phosphate, or magnesium hydroxide, PEG does not carry a risk for electrolyte disturbances, making it an ideal choice for elderly patients and/or patients with renal insufficiency.

CHAPTER 9

Endocrine Agents

AGENTS FOR DIABETES MELLITUS

What are the two general categories of drugs that are used to treat diabetes mellitus?

1. Insulin
2. Oral hypoglycemic agents

Which type of diabetes mellitus is each of the following statements referring to?

Loss of pancreatic β-cells	Type 1
Usually early onset	Type 1
Decreased response to insulin	Type 2
Ketoacidosis prone	Type 1
Usually adult onset	Type 2
Not ketoacidosis prone	Type 2
Absolute dependence on insulin	Type 1
May be controlled by diet and oral hypoglycemics alone	Type 2
Usually thin	Type 1
Usually obese	Type 2
Islet cell antibodies	Type 1
Near 100% concordance in monozygotic twins	Type 2

What types of drugs can elevate blood glucose concentrations?

Alcohol; β-adrenergic blockers; calcium channel blockers; combination oral contraceptives; diazoxide; diuretics; corticosteroids; lithium; niacin; phenytoin; sympathomimetics

What are the signs and symptoms of diabetic ketoacidosis?	Kussmaul respirations; fruity breath; abdominal pain; nausea; vomiting; polyuria; polydipsia; dehydration; fatigue
What chemical is responsible for causing "fruity breath" during ketoacidosis?	Acetone
What are the three ketones made during ketoacidosis?	1. β-Hydroxybutyric acid 2. Acetoacetic acid 3. Acetone
What is the term used to describe a rise in blood glucose usually between 4 and 11 AM due to the release of growth hormone, cortisol, glucagons, and epinephrine?	Dawn phenomenon. To determine the cause of elevated morning blood sugars, the patient must measure their glucose levels throughout the night. Then alterations in diet, medication doses, or medication choice may be made.
What is the term used to describe a rebound rise in morning blood glucose secondary to a low overnight blood glucose?	Somogyi effect. This usually results from hyperinsulinemia which decreases blood glucose. Glucagon is released when the patient becomes hypoglycemic, which causes a rebound spike in blood glucose levels. Decreasing the evening insulin dose is first-line therapy.
For each of the following types of insulin give the time of onset, peak effect, and duration:	
Aspart	0.17 to 0.33 hours; 1 to 3 hours; 3 to 5 hours
Lispro	0.25 hours; 0.5 to 1.5 hours; 6 to 8 hours
Regular	0.5 to 1 hours; 2 to 3 hours; 8 to12 hours
NPH (isophane insulin suspension)	1 to 1.5 hours; 4 to 12 hours; 24 hours
Lente (insulin zinc suspension)	1 to 2.5 hours; 8 to 12 hours; 18 to 24 hours
Ultralente (extended insulin zinc suspension)	4 to 8 hours; 16 to 18 hours; > 36 hours
Glargine	No peak; duration is 24 hours
Can insulin glargine be mixed with other insulins?	No
What is the most common side effect of insulin?	Hypoglycemia
What are the signs and symptoms of hypoglycemia?	Confusion; diaphoresis; tremors; tachycardia; seizures; coma; lethargy

Which sign/symptom of hypoglycemia is not masked by β-adrenergic antagonists?	Diaphoresis
What is the name of the incretin mimetic that increases insulin secretion, slows gastric emptying, and decreases food intake?	Exenatide
What is the name of the human amylin analog that is cosecreted with insulin and reduces postprandial glucose by prolonging gastric emptying time, reduces postprandial glucagon secretion, and suppresses appetite?	Pramlintide
What hypoglycemic agent is not contraindicated in a pregnant woman with diabetes mellitus?	Insulin
Other than blood glucose reduction, regular insulin can also be used for what condition?	Hyperkalemia. Insulin causes an intracellular shift of potassium. Insulin is given in combination with glucose to prevent hypoglycemia in this situation.

For each of the following oral hypoglycemic agents, state which drug class it belongs to?

Chlorpropamide	First-generation sulfonylurea
Tolazamide	First-generation sulfonylurea
Tolbutamide	First-generation sulfonylurea
Glyburide	Second-generation sulfonylurea
Glipizide	Second-generation sulfonylurea
Glimepiride	Second-generation sulfonylurea
Nateglinide	D-phenylalanine derivative
Rosiglitazone	Thiazolidinedione
Pioglitazone	Thiazolidinedione
Acarbose	α-Glucosidase inhibitor
Miglitol	α-Glucosidase inhibitor
Metformin	Biguanide
Repaglinide	Meglitinide
Nateglinide	Meglitinide
Pramlintide	Amylin analog
Exenatide	Incretin

For each of the following drug classes, give the mechanism of action:

Sulfonylureas

Block adenosine triphosphate (ATP)-dependent potassium channels, thereby depolarizing pancreatic β-cells which lead to insulin release (release mediated via calcium influx); insulin secretagogue

Thiazolidinediones

Bind to nuclear peroxisome proliferator activating receptor-gamma (PPAR-γ) which leads to increased sensitization of cells to insulin; decrease hepatic gluconeogenesis; upregulate insulin receptors

D-phenylalanine derivatives

Newest insulin secretagogue which closes the potassium channels on the β-cells leading to a rapid but short-acting release of insulin

α-Glucosidase inhibitors

Inhibit intestinal amylase and α-glucosidase causing a delay in the breakdown of complex carbohydrates into glucose which subsequently delays glucose absorption, thereby lowering postprandial glucose levels

Biguanides

Decrease hepatic gluconeogenesis; increase tissue sensitivity to insulin

Meglitinides

Nonsulfonylurea insulin secretagogue

Amylin analogs

Suppresses glucagon release, delays gastric emptying, decreases hunger

Incretins

Synthetic glucagon-like-polypeptide (GLP-1) analogs which potentiates glucose-mediated insulin release, decreases postprandial glucagon release, decreases gastric emptying, decreases hunger

What are the side effects of the sulfonylureas?

Hypoglycemia; cross-reaction with sulfonamide allergy; weight gain

What is the longest acting sulfonylurea?

Chlorpropamide

Which sulfonylurea can cause disulfiram-like reactions?

Chlorpropamide

Which sulfonylurea can cause syndrome of inappropriate secretion of antidiuretic hormone (SIADH)?

Chlorpropamide

The dose of what second-generation sulfonylurea should be decreased in patients with renal dysfunction?	Glyburide
The dose of what second-generation sulfonylurea should be decreased in patients with hepatic dysfunction?	Glipizide
What are the side effects of the thiazolidinediones (TZDs)?	Edema; congestive heart failure (CHF) exacerbation; weight gain; hepatotoxicity; macular edema (rare); increased bone fractures in women due to diminished osteoblast formation
Name two concomitant health conditions in which TZDs may not be used in a diabetic patient.	1. CHF 2. Liver failure
What are the side effects of the biguanides?	Diarrhea; lactic acidosis; decreased vitamin B_{12}; abnormal taste
What are the side effects of the meglitinides?	Hypoglycemia; upper respiratory tract infection
What are the side effects of the α-glucosidase inhibitors?	Abdominal cramping; diarrhea; flatulence
What drug with positive inotropic and chronotropic activity can be used to stimulate the heart during a β-blocker overdose?	Glucagon
Based on liver function test (LFT) results, when should therapy with a thiazolidinedione be withheld?	When LFTs rise above 2.5 times the upper limit of normal
What oral hypoglycemic should be withheld when the serum creatinine is above 1.5 for males and 1.4 for females?	Metformin
When used alone, can TZDs cause hypoglycemia?	No, TZDs do not cause hypoglycemia.
When used alone, can biguanides cause hypoglycemia?	No, biguanides do not cause hypoglycemia.
What time of day should meglitinides be given?	15 to 30 minutes before each meal

Would oral sucrose be effective in a hypoglycemic patient who is currently taking an α-glucosidase inhibitor?

No, it would not because sucrose is a disaccharide whose absorption is competitively blocked by the α-glucosidase inhibitors.

Would oral glucose be effective in a hypoglycemic patient who is currently taking an α-glucosidase inhibitor?

Yes, it would since glucose is a monosaccharides. α-Glucosidase inhibitors do not block intestinal transporters for monosaccharides.

AGENTS FOR DIABETES INSIPIDUS

What are the two types of diabetes insipidus?

1. Neurogenic
2. Nephrogenic

Which type of diabetes insipidus is characterized by insensitivity to vasopressin in the collecting ducts?

Nephrogenic diabetes insipidus

Which type of diabetes insipidus is characterized by inadequate secretion of vasopressin from the posterior pituitary gland?

Neurogenic diabetes insipidus

What types of drugs can cause a nephrogenic diabetes insipidus?

Lithium; demeclocycline; vincristine; amphotericin B; alcohol

What two effects does vasopressin have on the body?

1. Antidiuresis
2. Vasopressor

Where is the V_1 receptor found?

Vascular smooth muscle (causes vasoconstriction)

Where is the V_2 receptor found?

Renal collecting ducts (increases water permeability and reabsorption)

What is the drug of choice for neurogenic diabetes insipidus?

Desmopressin = vasopressin

What is desmopressin?

Synthetic analog of vasopressin with longer half-life and no vasopressor activity (antidiuresis properties only)

What is another name for desmopressin?

1-Deamino-8-D-arginine vasopressin (DDAVP)

How is desmopressin administered?

Intranasally; orally

What are the side effects of vasopressin?	Water intoxication; hyponatremia; tremor; headache; bronchoconstriction
What is vasopressin also used for?	Esophageal varices
What is desmopressin also used for?	Hemophilia A; von Willebrand disease; primary nocturnal enuresis
How is nephrogenic diabetes insipidus treated?	Thiazide diuretics in combination with amiloride; chlorpropamide; clofibrate
What drug that can cause nephrogenic diabetes insipidus is used to treat SIADH?	Demeclocycline *(ADH antagonist)*

AGENTS FOR THYROID DISORDERS

What are the signs and symptoms of hyperthyroidism?	Heat intolerance; nervousness; fatigue; weight loss with increased appetite; increased bowel movements; palpitations; irregular menses; proximal muscle weakness; moist skin; fine hair; hyperactive deep tendon reflexes; tachycardia; widened pulse pressure; tremor
What are the signs and symptoms of hypothyroidism?	Growth retardation in children; slowing of physical and mental activity; weight gain; cold intolerance; constipation; weakness; depression; dry skin; cold skin; coarse skin; coarse hair; bradycardia; muscle cramps; delayed relaxation of deep tendon reflexes
What are the signs and symptoms of thyroid storm?	High fever; dehydration; delirium; tachycardia; tachypnea; nausea; vomiting; diarrhea; coma
What are the two main active thyroid hormones circulating in the body?	1. Thyroxine (T_4) 2. Triiodothyronine (T_3)
Which thyroid hormone is more active in the body?	T_3 (up to five times more active)
What is the half-life of T_4?	7 days
What is the half-life of T_3?	1.5 days

What is the name of the enzyme that converts T_4 to T_3 in the periphery?

5'-Deiodinase (5 "prime" deiodinase)

What is the name of the enzyme that converts active T_4 to inactive reverse T_3?

5-Deiodinase

What is the drug of choice for hypothyroidism?

Levothyroxine (T_4)

When a hypothyroid patient is started on levothyroxine therapy, how long will the drug take to reach a steady state?

6 to 8 weeks

What are the adverse effects of levothyroxine?

Same effects as physiologic hyperthyroidism: heat intolerance; nervousness; fatigue; weight loss with increased appetite; increased bowel movements; palpitations; irregular menses; proximal muscle weakness; moist skin; fine hair; hyperactive deep tendon reflexes; tachycardia; widened pulse pressure; tremor

What biochemical marker is used to assess for adequate thyroid replacement?

Thyroid-stimulating hormone (TSH)

What antiarrhythmic agent can potentially cause either hypothyroidism or hyperthyroidism (more commonly hypothyroidism)?

Amiodarone (contains two iodine molecules)

To which three proteins in the blood are T_4 and T_3 bound extensively?

1. Thyroid-binding globulin
2. Thyroid-binding prealbumin
3. Albumin

The α-subunit of TSH is similar to the α-subunits of which hormones (gonadotropins) in the body?

Follicle-stimulating hormone (FSH); luteinizing hormone (LH); human chorionic gonadotropin (hCG)

What drug is used to ablate thyroid tissue?

Radioactive iodine (^{131}I)

What drug is used to treat cardiovascular effects seen in thyrotoxicosis?

Propranolol

What is a side effect of surgical removal of the thyroid gland?	Hypothyroidism almost inevitably results. Other possible complications include hypocalcemia due to removal of the parathyroid glands along with the thyroid.
What are the drugs of choice to treat hyperthyroidism?	Thionamides (propylthiouracil and methimazole)
What drugs inhibit the release of preformed thyroid hormone?	Iodide; lithium
What drugs inhibit the iodination of tyrosyl residues on thyroglobulin?	Propylthiouracil; methimazole
What drugs inhibit the coupling reactions that form T_3 and T_4?	Propylthiouracil; methimazole; iodide
What drugs block the conversion of T_4 to T_3 in the periphery by inhibiting 5'-deiodinase?	Propylthiouracil; propranolol
What are the side effects of propylthiouracil and methimazole?	Pruritic maculopapular rash; vasculitis; arthralgias; fever; leukopenia; agranulocytosis
Do propylthiouracil and methimazole cross the placenta?	Yes
What is the drug of choice for hyperthyroidism in pregnancy?	Propylthiouracil (more protein bound)
What drugs can decrease levels of thyroid-binding globulin?	Androgens; glucocorticoids; L-asparaginase
What drugs can increase levels of thyroid-binding globulin?	Estrogens; perphenazine; clofibrate; fluorouracil

ADRENAL STEROIDS

What are the three zones of the adrenal cortex?	1. Zona glomerulosa (outer) 2. Zona fasciculata (middle) 3. Zona reticularis (inner)

Name the steroid hormones produced by each of the following layers of the adrenal cortex:

Zona glomerulosa	Mineralocorticoids
Zona fasciculata	Glucocorticoids
Zona reticularis	Adrenal androgens

What is the major precursor of all steroid hormones?

Cholesterol

What is the principal mineralocorticoid?

Aldosterone

What is the principal glucocorticoid?

Cortisol, but note that cortisol does have some mineralocorticoid activity as well.

How do corticosteroids work biochemically in the body?

Bind to intracellular cytoplasmic receptors in target tissues then subsequently translocate to the nucleus where they act as transcription factors

What is the precursor of adrenocorticotropic hormone (ACTH)?

Proopiomelanocortin (POMC)

What chemicals are released when POMC is cleaved?

ACTH; lipotropin; β-endorphin; metenkephalin; melanocyte-stimulating hormone (MSH)

What drug is used to diagnose adrenal insufficiency?

ACTH (cosyntropin)

A cosyntropin stimulation test that results in no cortisol secretion characterizes which type of adrenal insufficiency?

Primary adrenal insufficiency (defect at the level of the adrenal gland)

A cosyntropin stimulation test that results in reasonable cortisol secretion characterizes which type(s) of adrenal insufficiency?

Secondary adrenal insufficiency (defect at the level of the pituitary gland) and possibly tertiary adrenal insufficiency (defect at the level of the hypothalamus)

What is the primary mechanism by which corticosteroids increase the neutrophil count?

Demargination, where the polymorphonuclear cells are detached from the endovascular wall and are therefore available to be counted in the peripheral blood smear

How is the production of arachidonic acid decreased by glucocorticoids?

Inhibition of phospholipase A_2

How is Cushing syndrome diagnosed?

Dexamethasone suppression test

Give examples of short-acting glucocorticoids:

Cortisone; hydrocortisone

Give examples of intermediate-acting glucocorticoids:

Methylprednisolone; prednisone; triamcinolone

Give examples of long-acting glucocorticoids:

Betamethasone; dexamethasone

Give an example of a synthetic mineralocorticoid:

Fludrocortisone

How long after initiation of glucocorticoid therapy does it take to suppress the hypothalamic-pituitary-adrenal (HPA) axis?

2 weeks

How should long-term glucocorticoid therapy be discontinued?

Taper regimen (taper regimen commonly used when discontinuing >2 weeks of glucocorticoid therapy)

How do you prevent suppression of the HPA axis while using glucocorticoids?

Alternate day dosing (every other day dosing)

List the adverse effects of glucocorticoids:

Acne; insomnia; edema; hypertension; osteoporosis; cataracts; glaucoma; psychosis; increased appetite; hirsutism; hyperglycemia; muscle wasting; pancreatitis; striae; redistribution of body fat to abdomen, back, and face

What drug inhibits glucocorticoid synthesis by inhibiting 11-hydroxylase activity?

Metyrapone

What drug inhibits the conversion of cholesterol to pregnenolone?

Aminoglutethimide

What antifungal can be used to lower cortisol levels in Cushing disease and may cause gynecomastia as an adverse effect?

Ketoconazole

What diuretic blocks mineralocorticoid receptors and also inhibits the synthesis of aldosterone and androgens (eg, testosterone)?	Spironolactone
What is the main side effect of spironolactone?	Gynecomastia; hyperkalemia
How does spironolactone work as a diuretic?	Antagonizes mineralocorticoid receptors in the kidney, thereby preventing sodium reabsorption in the distal tubules but not increasing potassium loss (therefore potassium-sparing)
Using an angiotensin-converting enzyme (ACE) inhibitor in combination with spironolactone can cause what major electrolyte abnormality?	Hyperkalemia
Name a potassium-sparing diuretic that does not have anti-androgen side effects:	Eplerenone, which has increased specificity for the mineralocorticoid receptor when compared to spironolactone

ANDROGENS AND ANTI-ANDROGENS

Is testosterone effective when administered orally?	No, as it is inactivated by first-pass metabolism.
What enzyme converts testosterone to dihydrotestosterone (DHT)?	5-α-reductase
Where is 5-α-reductase found?	Skin; epididymis; prostate; seminal vesicles
What drug inhibits 5-α-reductase?	Finasteride; dutasteride
What are the two main therapeutic indications of finasteride?	1. Benign prostatic hyperplasia (BPH) 2. Male pattern baldness
What are the uses of testosterone and its derivatives (danazol; stanozolol; nandrolone; oxandrolone)?	Male hypogonadism; increase muscle mass; increase RBCs; decrease nitrogen excretion; endometriosis (not first-line therapy for endometriosis given side effects)

What are the adverse effects of testosterone?	Edema; premature closing of the epiphysis; increased aggression ("road rage"); psychosis; increased low-density lipoprotein (LDL); decreased high-density lipoprotein (HDL); cholestatic jaundice; decreased spermatogenesis; gynecomastia; increased masculinization
What antifungal drug inhibits the synthesis of androgens and is also used as an antifungal?	Ketoconazole
What drugs act as androgen receptor blockers and are used in the treatment of prostate cancer?	Flutamide; bicalutamide
Which drug act as androgen receptor blocker and is used in the treatment of stomach ulcers?	Cimetidine (a histamine H_2-receptor blocker)
What is the mechanism of action of leuprolide?	Gonadotropin-releasing hormone (GnRH) agonist (daily administration suppresses LH and FSH secretion, thereby inhibiting ovarian and testicular steroidogenesis)
What are the therapeutic uses of leuprolide?	Prostate cancer; endometriosis

ESTROGENS AND ANTI-ESTROGENS—SELECTIVE ESTROGEN RECEPTOR MODULATORS

What is the major natural estrogen?	17-β estradiol
Where do conjugated equine estrogens (Premarin) come from?	Urine of pregnant mares
What is Premarin used for?	Vasomotor symptoms associated with menopause; vulvar and vaginal atrophy; abnormal uterine bleeding
Name two synthetic steroidal estrogens:	1. Ethinyl estradiol 2. Mestranol
Name one synthetic nonsteroidal estrogen:	Diethylstilbestrol (DES)

Mestranol is metabolized to what chemical compound?	Ethinyl estradiol
What are the therapeutic uses of estrogens?	Contraception; hormone replacement therapy (HRT); female hypogonadism; dysmenorrhea; uterine bleeding; acne; osteoporosis
How do estrogens affect serum lipids?	Increased triglycerides; increased HDL; decreased LDL
How is estrogen useful in preventing osteoporosis?	Decreases bone resorption
What are the adverse effects of estrogens?	Nausea; vomiting; headache; breast tenderness; endometrial hyperplasia; cholestasis; increased blood coagulation; increased endometrial cancer risk; increased breast cancer risk
Estrogen use is contraindicated in which settings?	History of or current deep vein thrombosis (DVT); history of or current pulmonary embolism (PE); active or recent stroke; active or recent myocardial infarction (MI); carcinoma of the breast; estrogen-dependent tumors; hepatic dysfunction; pregnancy
How do estrogens increase blood coagulation?	Decrease antithrombin III; increase clotting factors II, VII, IX, and X
What can happen to the female offspring of women who took DES during pregnancy?	Clear cell cervical or vaginal adenocarcinoma
How do estrogenic compounds work as contraceptives?	Suppresses ovulation
What does the enzyme aromatase do?	Converts testosterone to estradiol
Name three aromatase inhibitors:	1. Anastrozole 2. Letrozole 3. Exemestane
What are aromatase inhibitors used for?	Breast cancer
What is clomiphene used as?	Fertility drug

How does clomiphene work?

Antiestrogen that induces ovulation by inhibiting negative feedback of estrogen on the hypothalamus and pituitary (this suppression leads to increasing release of LH and FSH)

What are potential "adverse effect" of clomiphene?

Multiple births; hot flashes (10% patients); ovarian hyperstimulation (7% patients); reversible visual disturbances (2% patients)

What does SERM stand for?

Selective estrogen receptor modulator

Name two SERMs:

1. Raloxifene
2. Tamoxifen

What is raloxifene used for?

Prevention and treatment of osteoporosis in postmenopausal women

How does raloxifene work?

Estrogen receptor agonist in bone; estrogen receptor antagonist in breast and uterus

What is tamoxifen used for?

Breast cancer

How does tamoxifen work?

Estrogen receptor agonist in bone; estrogen receptor antagonist in breast; estrogen receptor partial agonist in uterus

Can tamoxifen increase endometrial cancer risk?

Yes, it has stimulatory effects on endometrial tissue.

Can raloxifene increase endometrial cancer risk?

No, it does not increase the risk of endometrial cancer because it has selective estrogen effects on the breast and bone but not the endometrium.

What are the adverse effects of tamoxifen?

Endometrial hyperplasia; hot flashes; nausea; vomiting; vaginal bleeding; menstrual irregularities

How does raloxifene affect serum lipids?

Decreases total and LDL cholesterol; no effect on HDL or triglycerides

What must you tell a female patient who is using hormonal contraception when she is given a prescription for antibiotics?

Antibiotics may decrease the effectiveness of OCPs; recommend the use of a "backup" contraceptive method in addition to the OCPs throughout the duration of the antibiotic course. This applies to both oral and intravenous antibiotics.

Which type of OCPs are used to shorten or suppress menstruations?

Combination OCPs

Which OCPs are used to palliate the effects of polycystic ovary syndrome (PCOS)?

Combination OCPs (often in combination with (oral) hypoglycemics)

PROGESTINS AND ANTIPROGESTINS

What is the major natural progestin?

Progesterone

What are the therapeutic uses of progestins?

Contraception; HRT (with estrogens); control of uterine bleeding; dysmenorrhea; suppression of postpartum lactation; endometriosis

Which progestins also possess androgenic activity?

Norethindrone; norgestrel

Why is progesterone added to a HRT regimen in a female with an intact uterus?

Decrease risk of endometrial cancer by preventing unopposed action of estrogen. If the patient is status post hysterectomy then combination (estrogen + progesterone) therapy is unnecessary.

How often is depot medroxyprogesterone given?

Every 3 months (13 wk)

How long does the levonorgestrel contraceptive subdermal implant last?

5 years

What are the adverse effects of progestins?

Edema; depression; glucose intolerance; breakthrough bleeding; increased LDL; decreased HDL; hirsutism (androgenic progestins); acne (androgenic progestins)

What drug acts as a progesterone antagonist and is used in combination with prostaglandin E_1 as an abortifacient?

Mifepristone (RU 486)

What are the adverse effects of mifepristone?

Abdominal cramping; uterine bleeding; pelvic infection; ectopic pregnancy

How do progestins work as contraceptives?

Prevents implantation of the early embryo into the endometrium; increases thickness of cervical mucus, thereby decreasing sperm access through the cervix

CLINICAL VIGNETTES

A 64-year-old man with a past medical history of hypertension, GERD, and type 2 diabetes mellitus presents to the emergency room with severe right upper quadrant pain. Acute cholecystitis is suspected and an abdominal CT with contrast ordered. Upon inspection of the patient's medication list, the attending physician orders one of the patient's medications to be held immediately and not resumed until at least 48 hours after the CT and adequate renal function has been ascertained. What medication was the patient taking that caused this concern?

The patient is taking metformin, a biguanide, for his diabetes. Metformin in combination with iodinated contrast materials can lead to lactic acidosis and decreased renal function. This is particularly concerning in patients who may already have some degree of renal impairment, such as diabetics. Additionally, preexisting renal impairment in combination with oral contrast can lead to increased serum levels of metformin, leading to toxicity. Therefore, it is imperative that the medication be stopped before use of the contrast medium and not restarted for 48 hours following the procedure. Proper kidney function needs to be documented as well before the medication is resumed.

A 24-year-old woman with no significant past medical history is being evaluated at a prenatal visit. Her husband accompanies her. The husband, who happens to be balding, quips with the doctor, "I know I look too old to be the daddy, but by the time the baby gets here I'm going to look ten years younger. I'm taking this great new medication that is making all my hair grow back." The obstetrician shows mild concern and asks exactly what medication the man is taking. What medication used to treat male pattern baldness must be avoided around pregnant women?

Finasteride, a 5-α-reductase inhibitor has been shown to be effective to treat some cases of male pattern baldness. Different formulations of the drug exist in various doses. Some patients will buy the less expensive brand of the drug and split the tablets to get the appropriate dose. This is a hazardous practice around pregnant females since even contact with crushed or broken tablets can lead to birth defects, notably abnormalities of the male external genitalia. In light of the potential adverse effects, the obstetrician could replace finasteride with topical minoxidil, which opens potassium channels and stimulates hair growth by an unknown mechanism.

A 19-year-old man presents to his primary care physician with complaints of increasing fatigue. He has occasional dizziness and feels weak. He believes recently he has contracted the flu because he has had nausea and vomiting, as well as muscle pain. He states that he has to be careful not to stand up too quickly, as this makes his dizziness worse. In-office evaluation reveals a thin adult male. Orthostatics are positive. The physician also notes a general darkening of the patient's skin, especially in the skin creases. Electrolyte tests are ordered. What other diagnostic test would be appropriate at this time, and what would be the likely results?

> The hyperpigmentation here is a red flag for Addison disease, or primary adrenal insufficiency. Decreased output of cortisol from the adrenals leads to a compensatory increase in corticotrophin-releasing hormone (CRH) from the hypothalamus, leading to release of POMC, the precursor of ACTH, from the anterior pituitary. POMC is cleaved into ACTH and melanocyte-stimulating hormone, thus leading to increased skin pigmentation in patients suffering from Addison disease. Decreased levels of the stress hormone cortisol account for the patient's other symptoms. To ascertain the primary nature of the disease, an ACTH (or cosyntropin) stimulation test should be ordered. A failure to produce an increase in serum levels of cortisol at either low or high doses of ACTH indicates failure at the level of the adrenal glands, or primary adrenal insufficiency. On physical examination, the hyperpigmentation of Addison disease may be distinguished from a suntan by examining areas unlikely to be exposed to sun, such as the axilla. Skin creases also tend to be darkly pigmented in Addison disease, as seen in this patient.

CHAPTER 10

Anti-inflammatory Agents and p-Aminophenol Derivatives (Acetaminophen)

Eicosanoids (inflammatory mediators) are synthesized from what chemical compound?	Arachidonic acid
Give two examples of eicosanoids:	1. Leukotrienes (LTs) 2. Prostaglandins (PGs)
How is arachidonic acid formed?	Phospholipase A_2 acting on cell membrane phospholipids
Corticosteroids block what part of the inflammatory pathway?	Inhibition of phospholipase A_2
Angiotensin and bradykinin have what effect on the inflammatory pathway?	Stimulation of phospholipase A_2
What enzyme acts on arachidonic acid to form LTs?	5-Lipoxygenase
Which LT is involved in neutrophil chemotaxis?	LTB_4
Which LTs are involved in anaphylaxis and bronchoconstriction?	LTA_4; LTC_4; LTD_4

What drug inhibits 5-lipoxygenase, thereby inhibiting LT synthesis?	Zileuton
What is zileuton used for?	Asthma; allergies
What two drugs act as LT receptor antagonists and are used in the treatment of asthma and allergy?	1. Montelukast 2. Zafirlukast
What are the adverse effects of zileuton and the LT receptor antagonists?	Increased liver function tests (LFTs); headache; Churg-Strauss syndrome
5-Lipoxygenase is found in which cell types?	Neutrophils; eosinophils; basophils; mast cells
Which LTs are considered the slow-releasing substances of anaphylaxis (SRS-A)?	LTA_4; LTC_4; LTD_4
What enzyme acts on arachidonic acid to form PGs and thromboxanes (TXAs)?	Cyclooxygenase (COX)
Where is COX 1 found?	Platelets; gastrointestinal (GI) mucosa; vasculature
Where is COX 2 found?	Sites of inflammation; brain; kidney; GI tract (low amounts vs COX 1)
Is COX 1 a constitutive or inducible enzyme?	It is a constitutive enzyme, meaning that its concentration is not influenced by the concentration of substrate in the cell.
Is COX 2 a constitutive or inducible enzyme?	It is an inducible enzyme, meaning that in resting conditions the enzyme is present in only trace quantities in the cell. Upon entry of the enzyme's substrate, the concentration of the enzyme increases exponentially.

Prostaglandin E_1 (PGE_1) does what to the following?

Patent ductus arteriosus	Maintains patency
Uterine smooth muscle	Increases contraction; used as an abortifacient during pregnancy
Blood vessels	Vasodilation
Gastric mucosa	Cytoprotective effect (inhibition of HCl secretion and stimulation of mucus and bicarbonate secretion)

What two $PGF_{2\alpha}$ analogs promote bronchiolar and uterine smooth muscle contraction?	1. Carboprost 2. Dinoprost
Why are nonsteroidal anti-inflammatory drugs (NSAIDs) effective in the treatment of dysmenorrhea?	Inhibition of PGE_2 and $PGF_{2\alpha}$ synthesis
What PGE_1 analog is used for impotence due to its vasodilatory effects?	Alprostadil
What is another name for PGI_2?	Prostacyclin
What are the actions of prostacyclin?	Inhibits platelet aggregation; vasodilation
What is the name of a prostacyclin analog and what is it used for?	Epoprostenol; pulmonary hypertension (HTN)
What are the actions of TXA_2?	Promotes platelet aggregation; bronchoconstriction; vasoconstriction
Increasing cyclic adenosine monophosphate (cAMP) will do what to platelet aggregation?	Decrease platelet aggregation (mechanism of action of PGI_2)
What is the mechanism of action of the nonselective NSAIDs?	Inhibit both COX 1 and COX 2, thereby inhibiting synthesis of PGs and TXAs
Name the three COX 2–specific inhibitors:	1. Celecoxib 2. Rofecoxib 3. Valdecoxib
Do COX 2 inhibitors inhibit platelet aggregation?	No
Which adverse effects of celecoxib have sparked debates about whether it should be pulled from the market or not?	Increased risk of cardiovascular events (myocardial infarction, stroke, and worsening of preexisting HTN)
What are the main therapeutic effects of NSAIDs?	Anti-inflammatory; analgesic; antipyretic; antiplatelet
What is the prototype NSAID?	Acetylsalicylic acid
What is acetylsalicylic acid also known as?	Aspirin; ASA

Does ASA act as a reversible or irreversible inhibitor of COX 1?

Irreversible

How does ASA irreversibly inhibit COX?

Acetylates serine hydroxyl group near active site of COX, thereby forming an irreversible covalent bond

What is the half-life of a platelet?

5 to 7 days

Why can't platelets produce more COX after ASA therapy?

Nonnucleated cells, therefore, lacking the capability of protein synthesis

What laboratory test is prolonged after ASA therapy?

Bleeding time

How does ASA work as an antipyretic?

Inhibits IL-1 stimulated synthesis of PGE_2 in the hypothalamus, thereby inhibiting alteration of the temperature "set-point"

Low-dose ASA does what to uric acid elimination?

Decreases tubular secretion (increases serum uric acid levels)

High-dose ASA does what to uric acid elimination?

Decreases tubular reabsorption (decreases serum uric acid levels)

What type of acid-base disturbance is seen in ASA overdose?

Mixed respiratory alkalosis with metabolic acidosis

Does ASA overdose cause an anion gap or nonanion gap metabolic acidosis?

Anion gap metabolic acidosis

What are the signs/symptoms of salicylism?

Decreased hearing; tinnitus; vertigo; nausea; vomiting; headache; hyperventilation; confusion; dizziness

Why is ASA not given to children especially during times of viral (varicella and influenza) infections?

Reye syndrome

What characterizes Reye syndrome?

Encephalopathy; hepatotoxicity

How can excretion of ASA from the urine be expedited?

Alkalinization of urine with $NaHCO_3$

What should be given instead of ASA to children with fever?

Acetaminophen (or acetyl-para-aminophenol, APAP)

What is the mechanism of action of APAP?	The direct fashion in which acetaminophen produces analgesia is unknown. The drug inhibits synthesis of PGs (via COX 3 inhibition) in the central nervous system (CNS), the only place in the body COX 3 is found. It also blocks pain impulse generation peripherally. Antipyresis is achieved via inhibition of the hypothalamic heat regulating center.
ASA can do what to asthmatics?	Exacerbate symptoms via bronchoconstriction due to unopposed production of leukotrienes
What is the "triad" of ASA hypersensitivity?	1. Asthma 2. Nasal polyps 3. Rhinitis
What is the mechanism of ASA-induced hyperthermia at toxic doses?	Uncoupling of oxidative phosphorylation
What are the GI adverse effects of NSAIDs?	Ulcers; gastritis; GI bleeding (via decreased PGs which act as GI mucosal protectants); nausea; abdominal cramping
If a patient is taking ASA and warfarin concomitantly, what should the dose of ASA be?	81 mg daily
ASA can do what to blood glucose?	Decrease blood glucose
What type of kinetics does ASA follow?	Zero order
Antiplatelet and analgesic effects of ASA occur at lower or higher doses than those required for anti-inflammatory effects?	Lower
What is the drug of choice for closing a patent ductus arteriosus?	Indomethacin
What is the mechanism of NSAID-induced renal failure?	Inhibition of PGE_2 and PGI_2 synthesis which are responsible for maintaining renal blood flow

Give examples of nonselective
NSAIDs other than ASA:

Ibuprofen; naproxen; diclofenac;
indomethacin; ketorolac; piroxicam;
oxaprozin; nabumetone; sulindac

What are the major differences
between nonselective NSAIDs and
selective COX-2 inhibitors?

COX-2 inhibitors have less antiplatelet
action and less GI adverse effects.

Which COX-2 inhibitors are
potentially cross-reactive in patients
with sulfonamide allergy?

Celecoxib; valdecoxib

Name two drugs that have antipyretic
and analgesic effects yet lack anti-
inflammatory and antiplatelet effects:

1. APAP
2. Phenacetin

APAP inhibits COX centrally,
peripherally, or both?

Centrally (inhibits PG synthesis in
the CNS)

Overdose of APAP can potentially
cause what life-threatening condition?

Hepatic necrosis

How is APAP predominantly
metabolized?

Glucuronidation; sulfation

Cytochrome P-450 2E1 metabolizes
APAP to which compound (this is a
minor metabolic pathway)?

N-acetyl-benzoquinoneimine (NAPQI)

Which metabolite of APAP is
hepatotoxic?

NAPQI

Which compound binds to NAPQI and
ultimately leads to its excretion?

Glutathione

What happens to patients taking APAP
when glutathione stores run out?

Accumulation of NAPQI with
subsequent hepatotoxicity

What drug is used to replenish
reduced glutathione during times of
APAP overdose?

N-acetylcysteine

What is the maximum daily dose of
APAP in patients with normal hepatic
function?

4 g per 24 hours

What is the maximum daily dose of
APAP in patients with abnormal
hepatic function?

2 g per 24 hours

CLINICAL VIGNETTES

A 16-year-old adolescent is brought into the emergency room by his parents who say that he tried to kill himself by taking all of the extra-strength Tylenol (acetaminophen) in their medicine cabinet 1 hour ago. Blood tests are ordered which return normal, including normal liver function tests. After 12 hours of observation in the emergency department (ED), the parents insist on taking their son home saying that he is obviously fine since he's been asymptomatic for so long. The father adds that there were not that many pills left in the bottle anyway, so the boy was just making a dramatic gesture. Besides explaining that their child needs a full psychiatric evaluation to ensure he is not a danger to himself and others, what other reasons should you explain to the parents regarding extended monitoring of the patient?

Acetaminophen toxicity has four phases. In the earliest phase, lasting up to 24 hours, patients may be largely asymptomatic and serum transaminases only begin to rise gradually approximately 12 hours after the toxic dose is taken. This is important to remember in patients who are exhibiting no signs of toxicity, even several hours after ingestion. As serum transaminases rise, right upper quadrant pain, nausea, vomiting, anorexia, jaundice, hepatic and renal failure ensue, ultimately with fatal results if the dose taken is high enough. Therefore, this patient needs to be closely monitored medically and N-acetylcysteine given to decrease mortality. The maximum daily dose of acetaminophen is only 4 g. When you consider that each extra-strength Tylenol Gelcap is 500 mg, even ingestion of a nearly empty bottle can have devastating consequences.

A 26-year-old woman is brought to the emergency room in respiratory distress. She is using accessory muscles to breath and appears tired. Auscultation of her lungs reveals wheezes bilaterally. Her husband relates that she has had a minor viral illness for the past 2 days associated with abdominal discomfort, vomiting, and diarrhea. She took Pepto-Bismol (bismuth subsalicylate) this morning to help her gastrointestinal issues. From what chronic medical condition does this patient likely suffer, and by what mechanism did the Pepto-Bismol cause her current symptoms?

Pepto-Bismol contains a salicylate, the class of medication to which aspirin belongs. Salicylates can cause bronchoconstriction in a small number (3%-5%) of asthmatics due to preferential production of leukotrienes via lipoxygenase from arachidonic acid when the cyclooxygenase enzyme is inhibited by the salicylates. Leukotrienes then contribute to inflammation of the respiratory mucosa leading to edema and respiratory distress. Therefore, asthmatic patients should be made aware of this rare, but potentially lethal side effect of all salicylate containing medications.

A term infant is born to a 29-year-old mother who has diabetes. Despite oxygen therapy, the infant develops increasing cyanosis in the hours following birth. The cyanosis is increased during crying spells. Transposition of the great arteries (TGA) is diagnosed. What medication should the infant be given before definitive surgical correction can take place?

TGA is more common in infants born to diabetic mothers. The great vessels are reversed in these patients so that the aorta arises from the right ventricle and the pulmonary artery arises from the left ventricle. Oxygenated blood cannot reach the systemic circulation in this fashion. At this point, the infant is being kept alive by the still patent ductus arteriosus, a connection between the aorta and pulmonary artery that allows the pulmonary circulation to be bypassed *in utero*. The ductus begins to close shortly after birth, normally within 12 to 24 hours. Closure will be fatal in this infant's case. Patency is maintained by prostaglandins. Therefore, prostaglandin analogs such as alprostadil or misoprostol should be used while awaiting surgery.

CHAPTER 11

Miscellaneous Topics in Pharmacology

IMMUNOSUPPRESSIVE AGENTS

What are the main targets of immunosuppressive agents?

Inhibition of gene expression; inhibition of lymphocyte signaling and activation; depletion of proliferating lymphocytes; inhibition of cytokine action; depletion of specific immune cells; blockade of costimulation; blockade of cell adhesion and migration; inhibition of complement activation

Which agents are signaling inhibitors of B-/T-cell proliferation?

Cyclosporine A, tacrolimus, and sirolimus

What is the mechanism of action of cyclosporine A?

Complexes with cyclophilin to inhibit calcineurin, thereby decreasing interleukin (IL)-2, which is the main inducer for activation of T lymphocytes

What are the main therapeutic indications of cyclosporine A?

Prevention of organ rejection in heart, kidney, and liver transplants

What are the adverse effects of cyclosporine A?

Nephrotoxicity; hepatotoxicity; cytomegalovirus (CMV) infections; hypertension; hyperkalemia; hirsutism; glucose intolerance; gingival hyperplasia; tremor; upper respiratory infections; anemia; leukopenia; thrombocytopenia

Name three medications that can cause gingival hyperplasia:

1. Cyclosporine
2. Phenytoin
3. Nifedipine

What major hepatic enzyme metabolizes cyclosporine A?	CYP 3A4
Cyclosporine A becomes more effective as an immunosuppressant when combined with what class of drugs?	Glucocorticoids
FK506 is also known as?	Tacrolimus
What are the main therapeutic indications of tacrolimus?	Prevention of organ rejection in liver and kidney transplants
What is the mechanism of action of tacrolimus?	It inhibits calcineurin by binding to FK binding protein (FKBP) rather than cyclophilin, cyclosporin's target protein. It inhibits the signaling pathway coupling cell receptor activation of IL-2 gene transcription (IL-2 synthesis).
What is the mechanism of action of sirolimus?	It blocks IL-2 receptor signaling required for cell activation and proliferation. It forms a complex with the immunophilin FKBP, it does not affect calcineurin activity, but inhibits the kinase mTOR, which is necessary for cell growth and proliferation.
What are the adverse effects of tacrolimus?	Nephrotoxicity; neurotoxicity; hypertension; headache; tremor; rash; hyperglycemia; hyperkalemia; anemia; leukocytosis; thrombocytopenia
Which murine monoclonal antibody interferes with T-lymphocyte function by binding to CD3 glycoprotein?	Muromonab-CD3 (OKT3)
Give examples of cytotoxic agents used in immunosuppressive therapy:	Azathioprine, mycophenolate mofetil, methotrexate, leflunomide, hydroxychloroquine, cyclophosphamide
Which cytotoxic agents used in immunosuppressive therapy are pro-drugs?	Azathioprine, mycophenolate mofetil, leflunomide
Which cytotoxic immunosuppressant is an alkylating agent?	Cyclophosphamide
Which immunosuppressant is a derivative of 6-mercaptopurine, antagonizes purine metabolism, and is cytotoxic to lymphocytes?	Azathioprine

Which immunosuppressant inhibits inosine monophosphate dehydrogenase, thereby inhibiting de novo guanosine nucleotide synthesis?	Mycophenolate mofetil
Which immunosuppressive agents are cytokine inhibitors?	Etanercept, infliximab, adalimumab, certolizumab, thalidomide, anakinra
Which cytokine inhibitor is not a tumor necrosis alpha (TNF-α) inhibitor?	Anakinra (It is an interleukin-1 [IL-1] receptor antagonist.)
Give two examples of immunosuppressive agents that inhibit costimulation:	1. Abatacept 2. Belatacept
Give two examples of immunosuppressive agents that block cell adhesion:	1. Natalizumab 2. Efalizumab
Give an example of an immunosuppressive agent that blocks complement action:	Eculizumab

AGENTS FOR OBESITY

What anorexiant works by increasing dopamine and norepinephrine levels in the brain?	Phentermine
What anorexiant works by blocking reuptake of serotonin, norepinephrine, and dopamine into presynaptic nerve terminals in the brain?	Sibutramine
What are the adverse effects of phentermine and sibutramine?	Tachycardia; hypertension; headache; insomnia; dry mouth; constipation
What drugs should be avoided in patients taking sibutramine?	Monoamine oxidase inhibitors (MAOIs); selective serotonin reuptake inhibitors (SSRIs); dextromethorphan
What popular name was given to the combination regimen fenfluramine and phentermine and why was it eventually pulled off of the market?	Fen-phen (combination of fenfluramine and phentermine); pulmonary hypertension and heart valve abnormalities. Fenfluramine was removed from the markets in 1997 in the United States because of these side effects.

What antiobesity agent inhibits gastric and pancreatic lipase, thereby inhibiting breakdown of dietary fat?	Orlistat
What are the adverse effects of orlistat?	Oily spotting; abdominal discomfort; flatus with discharge; fatty stools; fecal urgency; increased defecation
What vitamin supplementation is recommended in patients taking orlistat?	Fat-soluble vitamins
What are the fat-soluble vitamins?	A; D; E; K

AGENTS FOR OSTEOPOROSIS

Give examples of medications that belong to the bisphosphonate drug class:	Alendronate; risedronate; etidronate; pamidronate; ibandronate
What is the mechanism of action of the bisphosphonates?	Inhibition of osteoclast-mediated bone resorption
Which bisphosphonate can only be administered intravenously?	Pamidronate
What must patients be counseled on regarding oral bisphosphonate therapy?	Take medication with a full glass of water and stay in a sitting or standing position for 30 minutes following administration to prevent esophageal irritation.
Intravenous pamidronate can also be used to treat what conditions?	Hypercalcemia of malignancy; osteolytic bone lesions associated with multiple myeloma or metastatic breast cancer
What selective estrogen receptor modulator can increase bone density in women without increasing the risk for endometrial cancer?	Raloxifene
How is calcitonin administered?	Intranasally
What is the source of medically used intranasal calcitonin?	Salmon

How much calcium should a postmenopausal woman take daily?

1500 mg/d

Calcium should be taken with what other supplement to enhance its absorption?

Vitamin D

What recombinant N-terminal 34-amino-acid sequence of parathyroid hormone stimulates osteoblast function, increases gastrointestinal (GI) calcium absorption, and increases renal tubular reabsorption of calcium?

Teriparatide

AGENTS FOR ERECTILE DYSFUNCTION

What prostaglandin E_1 (PGE_1) analog is injected into the corpus cavernosum and causes increased arterial inflow and decreased venous outflow to and from the penis, respectively?

Alprostadil

What is the mechanism of action of sildenafil?

Enhances the vasodilatory effect of nitric oxide (NO) by inhibiting phosphodiesterase type 5 (PDE-5) which allows for increased cyclic guanosine monophosphate (cGMP) levels (cGMP causes smooth muscle relaxation in the corpus cavernosum)

Name two other PDE-5 inhibitors used in the treatment of erectile dysfunction:

1. Tadalafil
2. Vardenafil
3. Udenafil
4. Avanafil

What are the adverse effects of sildenafil?

Headache; dizziness; color vision disturbances; hypotension

Sildenafil is contraindicated in patients taking what type of medications?

Nitrates (potentiates hypotension)

AGENTS FOR RHEUMATOID ARTHRITIS

For the following disease-modifying antirheumatic drugs (DMARDs), give the mechanism of action:

Glucocorticoids

Decrease production of inflammatory mediators; suppression of neutrophil migration

Etanercept

Recombinant tumor necrosis factor (TNF) receptor linked to the Fc portion of human IgG1; binds TNF and inhibits its interaction with cell surface receptors

Infliximab

Chimeric monoclonal antibody that binds to human TNF-α, thereby interfering with its activity

Leflunomide

Inhibits dihydro-orotic acid dehydrogenase, thereby inhibiting pyrimidine synthesis

Anakinra

IL-1 receptor antagonist

Gold salts

Inhibit phagocytosis and lysosomal enzyme activity of macrophages

Methotrexate

Inhibits dihydrofolate reductase; increases adenosine levels (this is methotrexate's anti-inflammatory mechanism of action)

Hydroxychloroquine

Interferes with lysosomal function; inhibits chemotaxis of neutrophils and eosinophils

Penicillamine

Depresses circulating rheumatoid factor (RF); depresses T-lymphocyte activity

What is RF?

IgM directed against IgG

What other disease is penicillamine used to treat?

Wilson disease

What are the adverse reactions for the following DMARDs?

Glucocorticoids	Acne; insomnia; edema; hypertension; osteoporosis; cataracts; glaucoma; psychosis; increased appetite; hirsutism; hyperglycemia; muscle wasting; pancreatitis; striae; redistribution of body fat to abdomen, back, and face
Etanercept	Hypersensitivity; headache; local injection site reactions; respiratory tract infection; positive antinuclear antibody (ANA); activation of latent tuberculosis
Infliximab	Headache; rash; nausea; diarrhea; urinary tract infection; infusion reactions; arthralgia; upper respiratory infection; activation of latent tuberculosis
Leflunomide	Pregnancy category X; hepatotoxicity; rash; alopecia
Anakinra	Local injection site reactions; headache; infection
Gold salts	Nephrotoxicity; dermatitis; alopecia; eosinophilia; leukopenia; thrombocytopenia; hematuria; nausea; vomiting
Methotrexate	Mucositis; nausea; vomiting; diarrhea; nephrotoxicity; leukopenia; thrombocytopenia; hepatotoxicity; pneumonitis; crystalluria
Hydroxychloroquine	Cardiomyopathy; alopecia; visual disturbances; anorexia; nausea; vomiting; diarrhea; aplastic anemia; agranulocytosis; hemolysis in G6PD deficiency; cinchonism; exacerbation of porphyria
Penicillamine	Vasculitis; alopecia; hypoglycemia; thyroiditis; eosinophilia; hemolytic anemia; thrombotic thrombocytopenic purpura (TTP); hepatotoxicity; proteinuria

AGENTS FOR GOUT

What two categories do gout patients fall into pathophysiologically?	1. Overproducers 2. Underexcretors
Which drug is a xanthine oxidase inhibitor?	Allopurinol
What biochemical process is the enzyme xanthine oxidase involved in?	Purine metabolism
Which two drugs require dosage reductions when given concomitantly with allopurinol (because they are metabolized by xanthine oxidase)?	1. 6-Mercaptopurine 2. Azathioprine (reduce to 25% of normal dose)
What is the most common side effect of allopurinol?	Skin rash
Name other potential side effects of allopurinol:	Nausea; vomiting; renal impairment; acute tubular necrosis; agranulocytosis; Stevens-Johnson syndrome
Name three uricosuric agents:	1. Probenecid 2. Sulfinpyrazone 3. High-dose aspirin
Define uricosuric:	Enhancing renal excretion of uric acid
What is the mechanism of action of probenecid?	Inhibits proximal tubular resorption of uric acid
Probenecid inhibits the tubular secretion of what antibiotic and is sometimes given in combination to prolong its half-life?	Penicillin
How is acute gout treated?	Colchicine; nonsteroidal anti-inflammatory drugs (NSAIDs)
Why is allopurinol not used in the treatment of an acute gout attack?	May actually precipitate acute gouty arthritis and therefore perpetuate the acute gout attack (used for prevention and not treatment of gout attacks)

What is the mechanism of action of colchicine?

Increases depolymerization of microtubules; decreases leukocyte motility; decreases phagocytosis in joints and lactic acid production, thereby reducing deposition of urate crystals

What are the adverse effects of colchicine?

Nausea; vomiting; diarrhea; abdominal pain; agranulocytosis; aplastic anemia; bone marrow suppression; alopecia; myopathy; arrhythmia; hepatotoxicity

RETINOIDS

Retinoic acid shares a similar structure and function with what fat-soluble vitamin?

Vitamin A

13-cis-Retinoic acid is also known as what drug?

Isotretinoin (Accutane)

What is the major therapeutic indication of isotretinoin?

Acne

Isotretinoin belongs in what pregnancy risk factor category?

Pregnancy category X. This drug should not be used in pregnant patients under any circumstances. Fetal isotretinoin syndrome involves fetal craniofacial, cardiac, and CNS defects.

What is the mechanism of action of isotretinoin?

Decreases sebaceous gland size and reduces sebum production; regulates cell proliferation and differentiation; decreases hyperkeratinization; decreases androgen levels; decreases *Propionibacterium acnes* levels (bacterium associated with acne)

Hypervitaminosis A can damage what major organ?

Liver

All-*trans*-retinoic acid (ATRA) is also known as what drug?

Tretinoin

What is the major therapeutic indication of ATRA?

Induction of remission in patients with acute promyelocytic leukemia (APL)

What is the mechanism of action of tretinoin (when used for acne)?	Binds to nuclear receptors and inhibits clonal proliferation and granulocyte differentiation

HERBAL MEDICATIONS

Does the United States Food and Drug Administration (FDA) regulate herbal medications?	No
Are herbal medications considered "drugs" by FDA standards?	No, considered "nutritional supplements"
What herbal medication is used for migraine and fever?	Feverfew
What herbal medication is used for "jet lag"?	Melatonin
What herbal medication is used for depression?	St. John's wort
What herbal medication is used for benign prostate hyperplasia (BPH)?	Saw palmetto
What herbal medication is used for anxiety?	Kava kava
What herbal medication is used for Alzheimer disease?	Gingko biloba
What herbal medication is used for hypercholesterolemia?	Garlic
What herbal medication is used for the common cold?	Echinacea
What herbal medication is used for hepatitis?	Milk thistle
What herbal medication is used to treat hot flushes in menopause?	Black cohosh
Is St. John's wort a metabolic enzyme inducer or inhibitor?	Inducer

What herbal supplements should one use with caution when using warfarin concomitantly?

The G4 supplements: garlic, ginger, gingko, and ginseng. These substances may interact with warfarin, and some, especially gingko which has antiplatelet effects, may increase bleeding risk. Ginseng may decrease warfarin's effects.

SUBSTANCE ABUSE AND TOLERANCE

What are the physiologic effects of heroin?

Euphoria; decreased motor function; respiratory depression; miosis

What are some of the signs/symptoms of heroin withdrawal?

Nausea; vomiting; muscle aches; yawning; lacrimation; rhinorrhea; diarrhea; sweating; fever; mydriasis; piloerection; insomnia

What is another name for piloerection?

Goose bumps

How can heroin overdose lead to death?

Acute respiratory depression

What drug is used for the treatment of heroin abuse?

Methadone (μ-receptor agonist)

What drug is used to treat respiratory depression during an opioid overdose?

Naloxone

What drug is used to counteract the sympathetic effects of heroin withdrawal?

Clonidine

What is the mechanism of action of cocaine?

Blocks reuptake of dopamine, serotonin, and norepinephrine

What is the mechanism of action of amphetamines?

Ultimately, they increase the release of catecholamines from presynaptic nerve endings.

What are the physiologic effects of cocaine and amphetamines?

Euphoria; reduced inhibitions; reduced sleep; reduced appetite; tachycardia; sweating; increased alertness; pupillary dilation

What are the withdrawal signs/symptoms of cocaine and amphetamines?

Depression; increased sleep; increased drug cravings; bradycardia; dysphoria

What are the physiologic effects of marijuana?	Analgesia; increased appetite; impairment of short-term memory; antiemetic; altered perception of time and space; change in motor and postural control
What is the active psychotropic component of marijuana?	Delta-9-tetrahydrocannabinol (Δ^9-THC)
What medication is a synthetic form of THC formulated in sesame oil and is used as an appetite stimulant in AIDS patients and as an antiemetic during chemotherapy in cancer patients?	Dronabinol
What are the signs/symptoms of marijuana withdrawal?	Restlessness; irritability; agitation; insomnia; nausea
Is overdose of marijuana fatal?	No
Give examples of hallucinogenic drugs:	Methylenedioxymethamphetamine (MDMA; has hallucinogenic properties, yet is usually classified as a stimulant); mescaline; psilocybin; lysergic acid diethylamide (LSD); phencyclidine (PCP)
MDMA is also known as?	Ecstasy
Ecstasy can be neurotoxic to which type of neurons?	Serotonergic neurons
What is a major side effect of LSD?	Flashbacks
Is overdose of LSD fatal?	No
Does LSD have reinforcing effects?	No
What drug class does PCP and ketamine belong to?	Dissociative anesthetics
Is overdose of PCP fatal?	Yes, it is potentially fatal.
Does PCP have reinforcing effects?	Yes
What types of ocular disturbances are seen in PCP intoxication?	Vertical and horizontal nystagmus

TOXICOLOGY

Name the antidote for each type of poisoning:

Atropine	Acetylcholinesterase inhibitors
Arsenic, gold	Dimercaprol
Lead, mercury	Dimercaprol; succimer; penicillamine
Acetylcholinesterase inhibitors	Atropine with pralidoxime
Acetaminophen	N-acetylcysteine
Benzodiazepines	Flumazenil
β-Blockers	Glucagon
Copper	Penicillamine
Carbon monoxide	Oxygen (hyperbaric)
Digoxin	Digoxin immune Fab
Heparin	Protamine
Iron	Deferoxamine; deferasirox
Theophylline	β-Blockers
Warfarin	Vitamin K; fresh frozen plasma (FFP)
Thrombolytics	Aminocaproic acid; tranexamic acid
Opioids	Naloxone

What are the signs and symptoms of arsenic poisoning?

"Rice water" stools; GI discomfort; seizures; pallor; skin pigmentation; alopecia; bone marrow suppression; stocking glove neuropathy

What are the signs and symptoms of iron poisoning?

Bloody diarrhea; shock; coma; dyspnea; necrotizing gastroenteritis; hematemesis

What are the signs and symptoms of lead poisoning?

Nausea; vomiting; diarrhea; tinnitus; encephalopathy; anemia; neuropathy; nephropathy; infertility; hepatitis

What are the signs and symptoms of mercury poisoning?

Ataxia; auditory loss; visual loss; chest pain; pneumonitis; nausea; vomiting; renal failure; shock

What are the signs and symptoms of tricyclic antidepressant (TCA) poisoning?

Hyperthermia; coma; convulsions; cardiotoxicity; mydriasis; constipation; prolonged QT interval

| What are the signs and symptoms of SSRI poisoning (must be when used concomitantly with other serotonergic agents such as MAOIs or TCAs)? | Tachycardia; hypertension; seizures; hyperthermia; agitation; muscle rigidity; hallucinations |

CLINICAL VIGNETTES

A 66-year-old man with a past medical history of stable angina well controlled with oral nitroglycerin comes in for a regular check up to his primary care physician's office. After you politely ask about his wife he replies, "Well, she's not too happy with me lately." After some gentle prodding you elicit a history of erectile dysfunction. He asks you about a medication he saw on TV, Viagra (sildenafil). You inform him that because he takes nitrates he cannot also take this medication due to potentially fatal interactions. What alternative medication might you suggest for this patient?

The phosphodiesterase inhibiting properties of sildenafil cause vasodilation, allowing increased blood flow to maintain an erection. However, when used concomitantly with another vasodilating drug such as nitroglycerin, blood pressures may fall to levels insufficient to perfuse vital organs, especially in someone with preexisting heart disease. Therefore, an alternative agent must be used to treat this man's erectile dysfunction. Alprostadil is a less popular medication than sildenafil since it must be injected directly into the corpus cavernosa, but it does not have the systemic effects seen with sildenafil, making it a viable alternative to treat this patient's condition.

A 74-year-old woman undergoes a bone scan to evaluate her bone density. Her T-score comes back at −2.7. What is the mechanism of the class of medications that are first-line therapy for this woman's medical condition?

This patient has osteoporosis, defined as a T-score of less than −2.5. Studies have found the most benefit in early preventative treatment in women with the highest risk for fracture, that is, those with lower (more negative) T-scores. Bisphosphonates are generally first-line therapy for osteoporosis. Bisphosphonates work by binding to hydroxyapatite crystal in bone and inhibiting osteoclast-mediated bone resorption.

A 53-year-old man presents to your office with a warm, swollen right metacarpal phalangeal joint. He notes that this pain began suddenly, and is exquisitely painful. What are your options for immediate treatment for this man's pain, as well as long-term management for his condition?

This is a classic presentation of gout, seen most commonly in older men. It is caused by an accumulation of uric acid crystals in a joint or tendon. Acute management involves NSAIDs, colchicine, or steroids (local or systemic). Long-term management includes life-style modifications to decrease purine breakdown such as decreased intake of red meat and alcohol. Allopurinol, a xanthine oxidase inhibitor, may be helpful as well.

Common Drug Suffixes/Prefixes

Category	Suffix/Prefix	Examples
Opioids	-done	Methadone, hydrocodone, oxycodone
Local anesthetics	-caine	Lidocaine, prilocaine, benzocaine
Lipid-lowering drugs	-statin	Lovastatin, simvastatin
α_1-Adrenergic blockers	-zosin, -losin	Prazosin, tamsulosin
ACE inhibitors	-pril	Enalapril, ramipril
Thiazide diuretics	-thiazide	Chlorothiazide, hydrochlorothiazide
Angiotensin receptor blockers (ARB)	-artan	Losartan, valsartan
β-Adrenergic blockers	-olol	Propranolol, esmolol
Calcium channel blockers	-dipine	Amlodipine, felodipine
Low-molecular-weight heparins	-parin	Enoxaparin
Thrombolytics	-ase	Alteplase, urokinase, streptokinase
Benzodiazepines	-pam, -lam	Diazepam, midazolam
Barbiturates	-barpital	Phenobarbital, amobarbital
Antimigraine agents	-triptan	Sumatriptan, zolmitriptan
Bisphosphonates	-dronate	Alendronate, etidronate
H_2-receptor blockers	-tidine	Cimetidine, famotidine
Proton pump inhibitors (PPIs)	-prazol	Omeprazole, esomeprazole
Corticosteroids	-sone	Hydrocortisone, prednisone

Category	Suffix/Prefix	Examples
Bronchodilators	-terol	Albuterol, salmeterol
Cephalosporins	Cef-, ceph-	Cefazolin, cephalexin
Penicillins	-cillin	Penicillin, amoxicillin
Tetracyclines	-cyclin	Tetracycline, doxycycline, minocycline
Fluoroquinolones	-floxacin	Ciprofloxacin, moxifloxacin
Macrolides	-thromycin	Erythromycin, azithromycin
Antifungals	-azole	Ketoconazole, itraconazole
Antivirals	-vir	Ritonavir, tenofovir
Thiazolidinediones (TZDs)	-glitazone	Rosiglitazone, pioglitazone

Suggested Readings

DiPiro JT, Talbert RL, Yee GC, et al. *Pharmacotherapy: A Pathophysiologic Approach*. 5th ed. New York, NY: McGraw-Hill; 2002.

Gilbert DN, Moellering RC Jr, Eliopoulos GM, et al. *The Sanford Guide to Antimicrobial Therapy*. 36th ed. Sperryville, VA: Antimicrobial Therapy, Inc.; 2006.

Katzung BG, ed. *Basic and Clinical Pharmacology*. 11th ed. New York, NY: Lange Medical Books; 2004.

Koda-Kimble MA, Young LY, Kradjan WA, et al. *Applied Therapeutics: The Clinical Use of Drugs*. 7th ed. Philadelphia, PA: Lippincott Williams & Wilkins; 2001.

Physicians' Desk Reference. 59th ed. Montvale, NJ: Thomson PDR; 2004.

Index

Note: Page numbers followed by *f* indicate figures.